THE
MENOPAUSE
DIET

"A timely and much needed resource."
– *Foreword Magazine, 1999*

"Women should be eating this up!"
Ruth and Ed Shaw Radio Show, Talk America

"An invaluable book for really understanding how your body works on a hormonal level."
The Dance of the Soul Newspaper

"Not only is Larrian Gillespie a saint when it comes to helping women and understanding our too frequently unique health challenges, but she's also very, very funny! We call her "The Dave Barry of Menopause."
Carole Jacobs, Senior Editor, SHAPE Magazine

"I couldn't believe you could eat so much delicious food and still be on a diet. I can't wait to try some of them. I believe you have the perfect diet."
Tracee Cornforth, About.com's "Women's Health Guide"

"If you want to laugh your way through hot flashes, this book is for you."
Eagle Eye, Fall 1999

"Dr. Gillespie is to menopause what the Dali Lama is to spirituality."
Georgia Holt, mother of Cher, Academy Award winning actress

"Simply the best, healthiest, and wittiest way to lose weight!"
Mary Shomon, Author of "Living Well With Hypothyroidism: What Your Doctor Doesn't Tell You . . . That You Need to Know"

Amazon.com Customer Reviews:
This book is not about food punishment. Rather, it describes a flexible and satisfying way of eating that particularly suits the female metabolic and hormonal systems. The explanation of this diet makes great sense!

Within days of reading Dr. Gillespie's book my bloating has subsided and I am beginning to loose weight – not to mention how wonderful I feel – all this accomplished naturally by restructuring my eating habits.

THE MENOPAUSE DIET

Larrian Gillespie

Healthy Life
publications

Visit our website at
http://www.menopausediet.com

Healthy Life Publications Inc.
264 S. La Cienega Blvd., PMB #1233
Beverly Hills, Calif. 90211
1-800-554-3335
1-310-471-2375
1-310-471-9041 FAX

Publisher's Cataloging-in-Publication
Provided by Quality Books, Inc.
Gillespie, Larrian
        The menopause diet / Larrian Gillespie. – 1st ed.
        p. cm.
        Includes bibliographical references and index.
        ISBN: 0-9671317-0-7

        1. Menopause--Nutritional aspects. 2. Middle aged women--Nutrition. 3. Middle aged women--Health and hygiene. 4. Menopause--Complications--Diet therapy--Recipes. I. Title

RG186.G55 1999   618.1'750654
                        QBI99-582

First Healthy Life Trade Printing: September 1999
Second Trade Printing: February 2000

Printed in the U.S.A.

10 9 8 7 6 5 4

The information found in this book is from the author's experiences and is not intended to replace medical advice. The author does not directly or indirectly dispense medical advice or prescribe the use of this nutritional program as a form of treatment. This publication is presented for informational purposes only. Before beginning this or any nutrition program you should consult with your physician.

Inside cover photo: Robert Cavalli, Still Moving Pictures
Cover Illustration by: Carol Hoorman
Book Design by: Barbara Hoorman

dedication

To Alexian

Always my daughter
now too my friend

and my mother

Dorothy Olive Gillespie

contents

chapter

acknowledgments

A book is never done without the help of so many. I would like to thank Carole Jacobs for burning the midnight oil to edit this book, and Barb Hoorman for her creative styling. I hope you're proud of this book too!

To Elora Alden, for helping me get such a great shape. You make exercising fun!

I have been blessed with so many friends, without whom I may not have made it through many a dark time. To Georganne and Ebar, Cher, Georgia, Emma, Carol and Rosemary, Carol and Mike, Carol and Ray, Carole and Tom, Ali and David, Sharon and Lois, Marilyn and Don, Myra and Alby, Dave and Susan, Lynda and Wayne, CJ, Roy and Gene, Pat, Perry, Lois, Deirdre and Gregg, Annie and Jack, Cate and Cor, Helen and Richard, Helen, Kenn and Joanie, Christian, Gail and Grant, Jim and Anne, Cari and Kyle, Judy and Mike, Bud and Sandy, Fay and Norvel, Meredith and Shelly, Paula and Gerard, Füsun and Akif, thank you for showing me the meaning of unconditional love.

the menopause prayer

Oh God, grant me the hormones to forget the people I never liked anyway

The good fortune to run into the ones I do

And the eyesight to tell the difference!

menopause
a personal journey

Every woman must face the end of menstruation and fertility. But with it comes something NO WOMAN need resign herself to...gaining weight.

In my professional experience I had counseled women on hormone replacement therapy but put little emphasis on lifestyle changes. Yet I could see that well disciplined women going through menopause were gaining weight despite eating a "healthy diet." It was enough to make anyone cranky, let alone depressed!

All this had special relevance when it was my figure that began to change as I entered my forties. At first it was gradual, only a few pounds in six months, but within four years I had managed to pack an additional twenty five pounds onto my petite five foot two inch frame. I became an expert at "dress camouflage," emphasizing my newly developed bust line over my ever expanding waistline, while relegating my "older" clothes to the back of the closet. Large, oversize T shirts substituted as my new uniform while I filled drawers with belts that were no longer "fashionable" for me. What had once been a dancer's body had now morphed into a spider body—thin arms and legs attached to a large, round torso.

My day of reckoning came when I went for a physical examination and peeked at my report which frankly stated:

What had once been a dancer's body had now morphed into a spider body— thin arms and legs attached to a large, round torso

"Forty-five year old elderly multiparous white female, mild to moderately obese..." I wanted to scream!!! Me... OBESE!!! I knew what that meant. After all, I had written it about my very own patients. Obesity was next to slovenliness, carelessness...a glutton. How dare this man write that about me. Didn't he understand it was natural to gain weight when you go through menopause?

Women gain and lose weight differently than men

The truth hit me hard. I had become obese for my size. As a physician, I was fully aware of the health risks that came with being simply fat. But as someone who enjoyed food and the entire experience of preparing it, I looked forward to dinner, my only real meal of the day. As a surgeon, I skipped breakfast and avoided drinking fluids when I operated so I wouldn't be interrupted by nature's call and there was never enough time for lunch, as patients were waiting in the office. I rationalized every behavior deviation I knew contributed to weight gain, including blaming my mother for making me eat everything on my plate because there were "poor starving children in China." And then I realized if I didn't start putting my own weight loss on the top of my "TO DO" list, I was setting myself up for heart disease, diabetes, hypertension and years of disability.

This book is about my own personal journey through the process called menopause and how I lost the dangerous abdominal weight ALL women are prone to gain during this stage of life. In these chapters, I will reveal **why women gain and lose weight differently than men**, supported by the latest scientific research, and what you can do to avoid it. I will show you why women have been inadvertently fed the wrong information about diet during menopause and I will present to you explanations for these very natural symptoms and changes and what you can do about them. I will also share with you my perspective on current medical literature so that you can make your own intelligent choices about diet, exercise and hormone replacement therapy.

Over 60 million women are expected to be post-menopausal by the year 2000 and the latest longevity stats claim that anyone who reaches the age of 50 by the millennium has a one in two chance of living to 100. With these encouraging odds, no woman approaching menopause can afford to open herself up to the potentially dangerous health risks of "letting'er spread". With nearly 50% of American women age 45 and above classified as overweight, obesity has become a major health problem in the United States.[1] Although women live longer than men, they do so with more years of disability.[2]

It's time for a change.

chapter one
female, slim and sexy

Before me sat a woman in an oversize T shirt grasping her right side, sweating in pain while trying to suppress a belch. "Be suspicious of gallstones in anyone who is female, fat and forty" laughed my medical school instructor. But for this woman, it was no laughing matter. Menopause*, the time period that covers the ten years or more before the last menstrual period, is a critical span in a woman's life characterized by major biological and psychological changes which are important determinants of a woman's health in her later or post-menopausal years. While our ovaries kick out the last eggs in their stockpile, enzymes in our bodies, which are dependent on estrogen, begin to falter. Cholesterol levels start to climb, and the ratio of "good" versus "bad" lipids in our blood takes an abrupt nose dive, increasing our risk of heart disease and strokes. As if this wasn't enough, calcium begins to sneak out of our bones, leaving them vulnerable to everyday stresses while gallbladders go on strike, refusing to empty completely, spewing gallstones in their wake. This hormonal teeter-totter of life throws off our ability to burn calories and increases our sensitivity to glucose or sugar in foods.[4] And with that comes the inevitable weight gain of middle age.

The good news is you are not alone. Every

(*In clinical practice and medical literature, the term menopause is used extensively to describe the years immediately before and after the last menstrual period viz. the perimenopause or the climacteric.)[3]

woman over the age of 40 begins to develop changes in her body's ability to balance hormones against the control exerted by her nervous system. In fact, our nerves and hormones are so closely tied together they are known as the neuroendocrine system. Until recently, little importance was placed upon the interaction between our brain and hormones, but researchers are discovering that tissues thought to be inconsequential to our bodies may play critical roles in the fine tuning of our hormones, especially during menopause.

What I didn't know at the time was the role estrogen played in appetite control

As a physician who dealt with men and women's reproductive and urinary systems, you would think I'd know how to take proper care of my own body. Unfortunately, doctors are the worst patients. I never exercised, ate the recommended high carbohydrate diet espoused by the AMA, ADA and fashionable fitness magazines and relied upon my great genes to get me through life. And all was well until I turned 40.

I don't want you to think it was something dramatic that happened...far from it. Instead, it was insidious, like grey hair. Actually, I started turning grey, which I blamed on a harrowing episode with a patient who nearly died. Then I noticed my periods, which had always been irregular, were now every 28 days. At the same time, I began to develop an appetite. At first I thought it was just the result of my renewed interest in gourmet cooking, but when I could finish off an entire Lawry's Diamond Jim Brady cut of prime rib, complete with a giant baked potato and salad, I knew something was different.

What I didn't know at the time was the role estrogen played in appetite control. Recent research has implicated estradiol, the most potent and active form of estrogen, in the control of eating.[5,6] When estradiol levels drop, so does the release of cholecystokinin, a hormone produced by the pancreas which signals our gallbladders to empty. This in turn makes us feel full or satiated, especially when we have any saturated fat in our diet. During menopause, however, women begin to show a substantial delay in gallbladder emptying and just don't feel full as soon as they should.[7] As a result, portion size increases, and with that the number of calories consumed per feeding.

Changes in our ability to handle carbohydrates add another wallop. As blood sugar rises, so does our hunger quotient and any cholecystokinin released not only fails to signal we're full, but paradoxically increases our appetite.[8] So if you eat a high glycemic carbohydrate, such as popcorn with butter, you'll be even hungrier. Was it any wonder I could eat like a lumberjack! All this made me take a serious look at the changes menopause was having on my body, especially my stomach.

In order to appreciate how different things were becoming, it is important to learn how our digestive system works in the first place.

a trip through your digestive tract

Imagine your stomach is like a washing machine. You first "load" it with food, which has not yet been carefully sorted; that is, proteins, carbohydrates and fat all get tossed in together. Your stomach next adds the "pre-treatment enzymes" and detergent, called hormones. Gastrin stimulates the release of serotonin, histamine, hydrochloric acid and acetylcholine which cause the stomach to contract. The enzyme pepsin efficiently seeks out any of the aromatic amino acids in your food, that is tryptophan, tyrosine and phenylalanine, and chops them off from the rest of the proteins. The "cycle" changes and the emulsified food is now spun into the duodenum, or first part of the small intestine where a concert of actions take place under the direction of the pancreas. First chymotrypsin acts like a "bleach" to remove any residual "stains" or pieces of these same amino acids. At the same time, the pancreas signals your gallbladder to contract by releasing cholecystokinin, which makes you feel full. Carbohydrates and fats are broken down with the help of bile, which is stored in the gallbladder. The pancreas then releases insulin into the bloodstream to handle the sugars that have been extracted from carbohydrates, while the amino acids found in proteins are used to make neurotransmitters. When blood sugar starts to fall too low, the pancreas releases glucagon to prevent hypoglycemia. During all this time, the liver is directing your metabolism based upon the efficiency rating of your digestion. Finally, the pancreas ejects bicarbonate and "rinses" the food, stopping all the action of the stomach's enzymes while it performs the last cycle before sending it to the "dryer", the rest of your small bowel, where any excess water and tiny nutrients left over are absorbed into the bloodstream as the final cleanup from digestion. The entire cycle normally takes about two hours. (Figure 1)

Studies of women during menopause, however, show a distinctly different pattern of gastric emptying characterized by prolonged retention of food in the upper or first part of the stomach, preventing the timely release of cholecystokinin. Progesterone is the villain, exerting an antagonistic effect on the gastric nerves. Falling estrogen levels lead to complaints of an upset stomach and heartburn as excess progesterone relaxes the lower esophageal sphincter. This is especially noticeable at night, as lying flat in bed allows acid to flow back out of the stomach, irritating the esophagus. Interestingly, post-menopausal women **not** on hormone replacement therapy empty food at the same rate as men.

Not only does our stomach fail to empty on time, but this change in our digestion starts a domino effect on metabolism. Distension of the stomach occurs which sends stretch signals to nerves surrounding the bottom of the stomach. The gallbladder, in response, becomes sluggish, and doesn't empty completely. This prevents the complete emulsification of fats in our diet. When we eat cereals, oils, sugars and meat

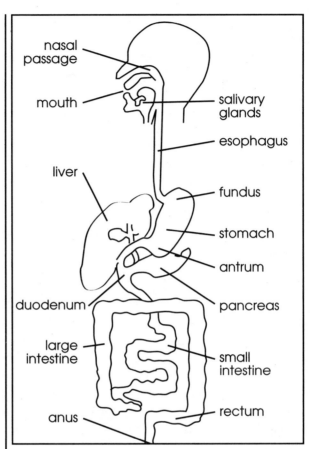

figure 1
the digestive system

instead of fish and fruits, we predispose ourselves to develop gallstones.[9] In a study of Italians, women who eat a low carbohydrate, high fiber diet and avoid alcohol have the least risk of developing gallstones.[10] A diet which limits calories to less than 2500 a day, decreases saturated fat and carbohydrates greatly reduces the risk of gallstones.[11]

The efficiency of our duodenal enzymes to break down food properly is compromised during menopause. As a result, our intestines are forced to handle incompletely digested particles, which exposes their delicate surface to damaging agents. Flatulence begins to develop as excess amounts of sugars, fats and amino acids ferment in the intestine. All this can lead to inflammation and even cancer.

It is not surprising that the stomach of meno-pausal women reacts more severely when infected with Helicobacter pylori, the infectious bacteria responsible for ulcers. While reproductive females are able to keep their immune reaction to a low level, women in menopause demonstrate weeping, destruc-tive inflammation of the fundus (first part) of the stomach and the antrum (lower part).[12] The delayed emptying allows the bacteria to remain in contact with the tissue for a longer period of time, increasing its virulence. Without the ability to properly stimu-late the release of cholecystokinin another hormone, somatostatin, is not produced to protect the stomach lining.[13] Like magic, you've created an ulcer.

A diet which limits calories to less than 2500 a day, decreases saturated fat and carbohydrates greatly reduces the risk of gallstones

our bodies not ourselves

If I'm honest with you, the ten years before we stop menstruating are the toughest on our bodies. As I told a patient, "Once the ovaries are dead, its easy. It's the dying that's the hard part!" There were days I swore my ovaries were threatening suicide. So let's look at the "risk factors" for an early menopause and the natural changes that occur during this time period.

In a study performed in Sweden, about 500 women who had been without a period for one year were studied in order to predict social and biological predictors for an early menopause.[14] Any woman who had a surgical or medical reason for menopause was excluded. Their findings were significant. **The more a woman smokes the younger she will be when her periods stop.** This is linked with a lower lung capacity, causing them to have less oxygen in their blood than their non-smoker associates. These same women also reported a higher degree of tiredness. It makes sense that if you can't get oxygen to the tissue, you'll cause cells to age more rapidly and die quicker. An anti-estrogenic effect of smoking has been suggested though the mechanism is not understood.

What is clear is that women smokers have less body fat, and that affects the blood levels of estrogens.

But these are not the only interesting discoveries. A later menopause is connected with a higher serum insulin and uric acid level. In fact, at the age of 40, a high insulin level is considered a marker for <u>normal</u> female sex hormone function and NOT for insulin resistance, as seen in post-menopausal women. So what does this mean? **As we age, our bodies begin to develop a sensitivity to carbohydrates as our estrogen levels start to fall, around the age of 40.** To understand the significance of this, let me explain what insulin has to do with our ability to metabolize carbohydrates.

carbohydrates and menopause

Let's start with a pre-menopausal female, that is, someone usually around 30 (remember, like everything, there are two ends to the bell curve and some women can be menopausal at 35). Carbohydrates are divided into two categories: complex and simple. It is perhaps easiest to think of these foods as starches and sugars which vary in the size of their particles. A simple carbohydrate has very small, fine particles, like sugar or refined, processed foods while complex carbs are more like raw, natural, large molecules such as lentils, squash and broccoli. In the course of "normal" digestion, it takes longer to absorb most large molecules because all food has to be broken down into the smallest particle. That is why small, simple carbohydrates get into your blood stream the fastest. However, some complex carbohydrates contain more natural sugar and can be quicker to get into the blood, such as corn, acting like a simple carbohydrate in triggering your body's insulin response.

Glucose is the fuel which enables the mitochondria to act like a thermonuclear reactor, splitting off electrons which generate energy for cellular function. Most importantly, every organ in our body requires glucose to function. Glucose is either used immediately as your cell's energy source or stored in the form of glycogen in the liver and in muscle as emergency reserves. **Once these sites are full, the rest is stored as fat.** The role of insulin is to keep blood glucose levels from rising too high by shoving glucose, amino acids and free fatty acids from the bloodstream as quickly as possible into every cell for immediate use. Like a teeter-totter glucagon, another hormone, prevents insulin from being too efficient and causing hypoglycemia. Both hormones are secreted by the pancreas. When we eat carbohydrates, the petite particles are absorbed from the small intestine into our bloodstream and we have an elevated glucose level. Like the newest vacuum cleaner, insulin "beats, it sweeps, it cleans" our blood of glucose by shoving it into cells, then storing any excess in fat cells. As if to add insult to injury, insulin signals previously stored fat to stay put while excess free fatty acids are then sent to the liver where they are converted into cholesterol.

Glucagon, on the other hand, is stimulated by proteins and a lowering glucose level and has the laudable job of promoting the breakdown of stored fat in order to achieve equilibrium. This is a GOOD thing! It's also capable of aiding the liver in converting amino acids derived from protein into glucose in case of starvation. The exciting news is that once glucagon levels are elevated, they remain so for at least four hours.[15]

menopause-dependent changes

As you can tell, our bodies undergo a lot of changes during menopause, the most significant of which may be alteration in our sensitivity to insulin. As estrogen decreases, thyroid levels begin to drop while insulin loses its effectiveness in lowering our blood sugar. This causes our pancreas to have to work overtime putting out more than the usual amount of insulin to do the same job. You already know that insulin aids in storing fat. This makes it MORE efficient at storing the excess glucose as fat as it becomes LESS efficient at lowering our blood glucose levels. An increase in body mass occurs. In short...we start to become fat. In fact, a specific syndrome, called Metabolic Syndrome X, has been identified in menopausal women. It is characterized by women who have two or more of the following conditions: insulin resistance with resulting elevated insulin levels, elevated lipids (especially triglycerides), obesity, coronary artery disease and hypertension. Not surprisingly, it has been found to be associated with estrogen deficiency.[16,17]

Statistics indicate that 34% of white women, almost 50% of African American women and 48% of Hispanic women are overweight.[1] Obesity is respon-sible for hypertension, gallstones, endometrial, kidney and breast cancer, heart attacks and diabetes, just to name a few diseases that can be modified or even prevented by losing as little as 5-10 pounds.[18-24] As women, we simply can't afford to trivialize the impact obesity has on our health. Although there has been a increase in the frequency of articles on menopause in the past 15 years, little emphasis has been placed on aging, stress, life-style changes, exercise or diet.[25] As you will see in the following chapters, each of these factors form an essential part in helping us stay slim and sexy at any age!

Obesity is responsible for hypertension, gallstones, endometrial, kidney and breast cancer, heart attacks and diabetes

chapter two

*buddha belly
syndrome:
the hidden danger*

Scientists are only now discovering that a healthy weight is not defined by the numbers on a scale, but by where fats are stored in the body. More importantly, not all fat cells behave alike, with the most metabolically active ones hiding like some creature in the dark deep inside the abdomen. As a result, you can be simultaneously very fit but fairly fat. Genetics plays a role in this, but scientists are acknowledging that menopause dictates where women put on fat after 40.

fat's gotten under your skin

Both visceral and subcutaneous fat have the same composition—75% fatty acids and 25% glycerol, a type of alcohol. While the fat cells **inside** our abdomen are smaller than their distant cousins on our hips, these little creatures are more active, releasing fatty acids into the blood stream while picking up additional fat for storage. Because they can snuggle up to the blood vessels surrounding all our internal organs, they can deliver fatty acids to tissue with little constraint. This means the liver is bathed with blood that is very high in free fatty acids, which results in less of the good cholesterol, called high density lipoproteins (HDL) and more of the bad or low density cholesterol (LDL). Any tissue surrounded by fatty acids is less able to remove insulin from the bloodstream, which results in increased fat storage. The more intra-abdominal fat, the higher the insulin levels.[26]

the omentum

As a surgeon, I constantly encountered the omentum, a fatty apron of tissue that performs the function of a barrier between the lining of the abdomen and the bowel in order to prevent adhesions. This organ acts as a giant sponge within your stomach soaking up any fluid in contact with it...blood, electrolyte solutions, lymph or fluid from ovarian cysts. It has the additional ability to concentrate neurochemicals, especially norepinephrine, epinephrine and dopamine from the GI tract in its venous blood and tissue.[27] This makes it a very active biological organ, capable of mobilizing fat in response to insulin and cortisol. This organ is able to swell and enlarge when faced with excess amounts of these neurotransmitters, which are found in red meat and manufactured from foods high in the amino acids tryptophan, tyrosine and tyramine. If you've ever eaten a meal and felt the uncomfortable tug of your belt before you left the table, it's your omentum working overtime. (Figure 2)

The more intra-abdominal fat, the higher the insulin levels

the rules of fat distribution

The regulation of fat distribution is a highly complex process, entailing profound effects on metabolism. By measuring the turnover of fat tissue triglycerides, researchers were able to show that fats are first stored in the omentum and retroperitoneal areas (the deep parts of your pelvis), then the subcutaneous regions of the abdomen and finally in the sub-cutaneous femoral area on the thigh.[28] In premenopausal women subcutaneous abdominal fat has a higher turnover than femoral fat tissue, a difference that disappears with menopause and is restored by estrogen. With abdominal fat, multiple hormone

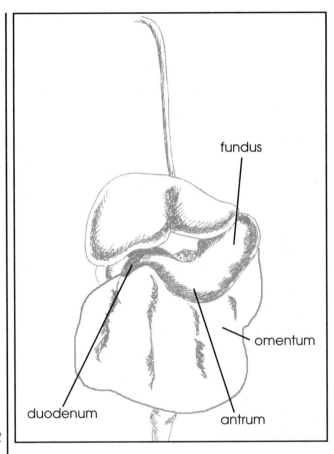

fundus

omentum

duodenum

antrum

figure 2

changes are found including elevated cortisol and male sex hormones in women, due to the information highway connecting the hypothalamus, pituitary and adrenals. Fat cells, under the direction of cortisol and insulin, promote fat storage by expressing lipoprotein lipase, a fat accumulating enzyme. Abdominal fat cells pack more in per square inch, and have a greater blood supply along with more nerve connections to detour fats to their area. In short, the balance between the fat accumulating couple (cortisol and insulin) and the fat mobilizing couple (estrogen and growth hormone) is shifted in favor of the former in menopause, polycystic ovarian syndrome, aging, depression, smoking and excess alcohol intake.

location location location

Like real estate, everything about fat boils down to its location. Fat cells, called adipocytes, have limits on how much fat they can store dependent upon their position in the body. Intra-abdominal or visceral cells are the sumo wrestlers of fat storage, enlarging to gargantuan size when we put our bodies under chronic stress. These lard buckets have more receptors for glucocorticoids than peripheral fat cells, allowing them to preferentially direct the fat traffic to their sites.[29] Insulin causes fluid retention by making us more sensitive to salt and expands the tissue surrounding these cells. Cortisol speeds up the intestine's ability to transport fat and this makes it harder for fat depots to clear out glycerol and free fatty acids, the products of fat breakdown, which prevents further mobilization of fat.[30] You can almost hear those fat cells squishing when you chomp down on a "stress relieving" bag of potato chips.

Insulin causes fluid retention by making us more sensitive to salt and expands the tissue surrounding these cells

the sensitive side of fat

Abdominal fat has a significantly stronger relationship with insulin sensitivity than peripheral non-abdominal fat, making women with the Spider Body shape more insulin resistant than those with fat on their thighs.[26] Scientists say abdominal fat may be a major reason why women develop insulin resistance.

With central obesity there is an increased risk for breast and endometrial cancer due to elevated levels of circulating estrogens created from alterations of male sex steroids or androgens in fat tissue combined with decreased levels of sex hormone-binding globulin (SHBG).[31] As insulin levels go up, the ovaries increase the production of male sex hormones—testosterone and androstenedione—and infertility occurs.[32,33] Meals high in carbohydrates stimulate higher levels of insulin which in turn causes a rise in androgens. Obese women with infertility are probably stimulating their disease process with every meal they eat. The great news is all this can be reversed by simply losing weight.[34]

The bad news is even a normal weight can be unhealthy in some women. Scientists measured the hidden fat within the abdomen of normal weight women by computerized tomography, or a CAT scan. Using a body mass index (BMI) of 25 as normal, they were able to determine that women aged 40 and above who had not completed menopause should have a desirable waist measurement less than 31 1/2 inches. If you are post-menopausal, you should strive for less than 29 1/2 inches if you don't want to raise your risk factors for heart disease and diabetes.[35] The swing of the needle on a scale means very little if you stuff your abdomen with most of your fat.[26]

the chinese connection

The significance of this information crosses all cultural lines. Studies on healthy Chinese men and women who had heavy upper bodies were at a higher risk of cardiovascular disease even though they weren't technically fat.[36] Deep intra-abdominal fat correlated with higher blood pressure, glucose, triglyceride and low HDL levels - all known to put us at increased risk for heart disease. So even eating a traditional oriental diet can't change the impact central body fat has on our survival.

After reading this research, I knew I could no longer justify the "Buddha Belly" I had acquired. My father died of a sudden, unexpected heart attack and his parents and brothers as well. I had inherited their body shape and genetics, but I was determined to prevent my genes from controlling my destiny.

how body shape can predict health problems

All women are NOT created equal when it comes to the shape of our bodies, as anyone knows whose stood in the open changing room at Loehmann's. Some women are pear shaped, with "saddle bag" thighs and buttocks, while others carry most of their "pot" on the belly and upper hips. But did you know that where you put on fat is directly under the control of your hormones?

hormones: fat dictators

During our childbearing years, estrogen directs fat to be stored on our hips and thighs as a quick access site for energy during breast-feeding. Physicians refer to this shape as a "gynecoid" or feminine figure. (Figure 3A) Once our estrogen levels start to drop during menopause, we no longer prefer our legs as storage sites for fat and we start hoarding blubber under the skin and within the abdomen. This gives us

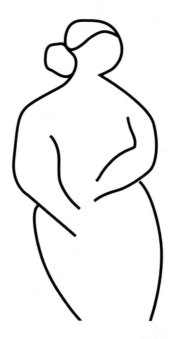

figure 3A
*gynecoid
shape*

a different body shape, called "android", which makes us look more like a man. (Figure 3B) This change is brought about by age, plain and simple. Growth hormone, which directs our fat metabolism and helps to build muscles, takes an elevator ride to the basement and we start to lose fat burning muscle mass. Once this happens our ability to burn calories falls and any excess food that finds its way down our digestive tracts gets sidelined into fat.[18,37] As we replace lean muscle with fat, we keep lowering our energy efficiency rating. Total body weight goes up and that's when the problems really start.

Hormones rule our bodies. I know you don't like to hear this but it's true. The amazing part is how something as simple as fat can start a chain reaction that will send our entire bodies spiraling into hormone hell.

insulin: the evil twin

When we gain fat a not-so-funny thing happens to our insulin levels - they go up - and that results in

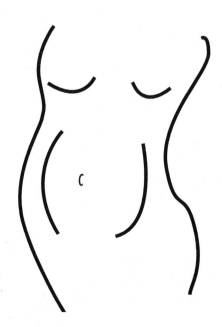

figure 3B
*android
shape*

more fat storage. It seems insulin can act like an evil twin, lowering our blood sugar when present in small amounts (the GOOD twin) but let it hang around for a while and it turns us into porkers. Progesterone, another hormone that helps us to hold onto a pregnancy in our fertile years, stimulates the pancreas to secrete insulin, and the more insulin in circulation, the more hostile our tissue becomes to its action of lowering glucose in our blood.[38,39] Cholesterol levels go up and the concentration of the good triglycerides goes down. High, sustained insulin levels accelerate the formation of blood clots, and that makes us more susceptible to strokes and heart attacks. As a final kick in the pants, it stiffens our blood vessels, causing hypertension.

High, sustained insulin levels accelerate the formation of blood clots, and that makes us more susceptible to strokes and heart attacks

the apple and the pear: it's not the garden of eden

So how do you tell if you have an apple or pear shaped body? The most reliable indicator seems to be your waist-to-hip ratio (WHR) followed by the circumference of your waist. To find your WHR, measure around the fullest part of your buttocks (this is your hip measurement) and then measure your waist (the narrowest part of your torso between your lowest rib and your iliac crest or hip bone.) Simply divide your waist by your hip measurement. A healthy ratio is less than .8 with an ideal ratio around .74. A WHR greater than 0.85 is characteristic of upper body obesity. Women with this android or male body shape have more bloated fat cells, higher sustained insulin levels, which become less effective at lowering their blood sugar, and are often producing large amounts of male sex hormones. In addition, they have elevated plasma lipid profiles and are at a high risk of developing non-insulin dependent diabetes.[40]

According to a study published in JAMA, women with a WHR of 0.76 or higher or a waist circumference of 30 inches or greater have more than a 2-fold higher risk of coronary heart disease.[41] Further studies show that women who gain weight in their abdomen have a higher risk of developing heart disease than those who gain weight in their legs.[42] So what is directing all these changes during menopause? A wedge-shaped gland called the hypothalamus.

this is your brain on patrol

Located at the base of the third ventricle in the brain, the hypothalamus acts as the "Great and Wonderful Wizard" of our hormones sending signals to the pituitary which in turn shouts orders to the other endocrine glands - the adrenals, thyroid and ovaries. (Figure 4) As our supply of eggs decreases, information is sent back to the hypothalamus informing it of an upcoming shortage in estrogen. This makes it a little hypersensitive - okay, plain cranky - and it begins to order the adrenal glands to swell, or hypertrophy in order to produce an alternate pathway for estrogen production. Once the adrenals swing into action cortisol, the stress hormone, gets released and fat cells open up to take on more storage. The amount of fat metabolism changes dramatically and those fat cells which have a greater blood supply turn into gluttons. Unfortunately, these are the very ones that surround the bowel and line our abdominal cavity giving us the android shape.

Women who gain weight in their abdomen have a higher risk of developing heart disease than those who gain weight in their legs

the threat to your health

Diabetes strikes over 8 million people, while an additional 8 million remain undiagnosed with non-insulin dependent diabetes (NIDDM or type II).[43] Astonishingly, an estimated 20 million persons meet the criteria for impaired glucose tolerance, a condition in which blood glucose levels are higher than normal but not high enough to be diagnosed as diabetes. Hyperglycemia and impaired glucose

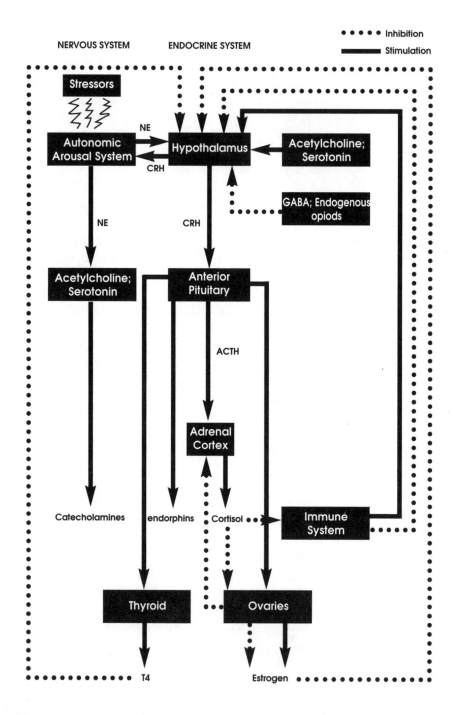

figure 4

tolerance, as seen with menopause, convey a significant risk for heart disease and full-blown diabetes.[44] Not surprisingly, it's the sugar extracted by our stomach from the foods we eat that results in the high glucose levels seen after eating in early undiagnosed diabetes. In fact, the first sign of diabetes is elevated glucose for several hours after a meal.[45]

Coronary artery disease kills more women, nearly 500,000 annually, than all cancers combined.[46] Women with heart disease are also more likely to suffer from diabetes, hypertension and high cholesterol levels than men. After menopause, the chance of dying from a heart attack in women nearly equals those of men. A postmenopausal woman has a 31% lifetime mortality risk from heart disease in contrast to a 2.8% risk of dying from a hip fracture or breast cancer.[47] As many as 1 in 8 women aged 45 to 54 has clinical evidence of heart disease. You've probably already guessed the two most significant risk factors for developing either diabetes or heart disease—smoking and abdominal obesity.

and now for the spider body awards

So what are the risk factors for gaining abdominal or central fat? In a study done by the American Cancer Society, women who eat large amounts of saturated fat, especially from meat, frequently drink alcohol, smoke, have multiple pregnancies or have gained a lot of weight since the age of 18 have twice as much chance of winning the "Spider Body Award" than women who eat a diet high in vegetables, exercise, complete menopause and take estrogen faithfully.[48]

Gaining weight during menopause does more than make you look fat—it can endanger your health, shorten your life span and even trigger life-threatening diseases. Now for the good news. If you look at all the illnesses listed in Table 1, **each and every one** can be modified by losing this dangerous abdominal fat.

If you're ready to change your lifestyle and want to be healthy for the next fifty years, let me show you how simple it is to lose the weight and keep it off. You don't need pills or surgery and you can end up saving a lot of money. Interested? Then let's get started.

Table 1

---

intra-abdominal fat as a risk factor

- Arthritis
- Hypertension
- Cancer of the breast, endometrium, kidneys
- Incontinence
- Coronary Heart Disease
- Kidney failure
- Chronic lung disease
- Kidney stones
- Diabetes
- Polycystic ovarian disease
- Gallstones
- Sleep apnea
- Stroke

chapter three
the menopause diet

It seems like your worst nightmare. After days of dieting and yes, even starvation, you sneak up on the bathroom scale like a stealth bomber only to discover you're still no thinner! According to Prevention, the world's largest health magazine, weight gain is the number one complaint of women in menopause whether or not they take hormones.[49] How food affects hormones is the focus of dietary endocrinology and scientists are only now starting to assess why women gain and lose weight differently than men.

It's a scientific fact. Women's stomachs respond differently than men's when digesting a meal. Numerous studies agree that we take almost an hour longer than men to empty our stomachs due to the effect of progesterone on the motility of the antrum, or lower portion of the stomach.[50] As a result, we are much more efficient at grabbing every little bit of carbohydrate from the foods we eat before we digest protein and fat.[51] This causes a more sustained rise in insulin, which increases our ability to store fat. In fact, our blood insulin and glucose levels can stay high for up to five hours after a 500 to 1000 calorie meal. This can set the stage for heart disease, hypertension, obesity, cataracts and the signs of aging.

This delayed but prolonged rise in insulin and glucose in response to carbohydrates inhibits the release of glucagon, the hormone that helps us to burn previously stored fat. In normal people, (they mean men...bear with me) within thirty minutes of eating protein, glucagon levels start to rise, peaking at two hours.[52] In fact, glucagon can stay elevated in blood for several hours after a protein rich meal. This gives your body plenty of time to use the fat around your waist and hips as the energy source to fuel your brain.

all carbohydrates are not created equal

Women's stomachs respond differently than men's when digesting a meal

Since 1927, scientists have known that different carbohydrates with the same nutrient composition produce different glucose responses in the body.[53] A "sugar profile" was developed for each food enabling doctors to predict the effect of digestion on the availability of glucose in the body. By comparing other foods to the glucose response which you achieve by eating just a few slices of white bread, a glycemic index of carbohydrate metabolism was established.[54-56] This gave doctors the freedom to exchange carbohydrate choices for diabetic patients without risking big swings in their blood glucose levels.

Not all foods, however, are created equal. The particle size of a particular food and the degree of gelatinization which it undergoes when cooked affects how much glucose or sugar can be obtained by digestion. Rice is a good example of a food that can vary markedly depending upon the amylose content. The higher the amylose, the greater the gelatinization and the lower the glycemic index (GI).[57] The more processed a food becomes, the smaller the particle size and the greater the GI. That's why bread, french fries, corn chips, canned pea soup, angel food cake and Cheerios™ have almost identical GI values and insulin responses.[58]

are women unique?

When it comes to measuring blood glucose responses, women are definitely unique. A standard glucose tolerance test extends over 2-4 hours, while in diabetic patients and women in menopause, 3-5 hours are needed to get a complete profile.[59,60] All this has to do with the rate of digestion. Like diabetics, women add an additional hour onto digestion because they are unable to move food from the bottom or antral portion due to delays in activating the sympathetic nerves which stimulate the stomach to empty. As a result, women and diabetics have a slower rise in the glucose and insulin response to food and these levels can remain slightly above fasting for several hours.[61] Since our bodies were designed to feed "two" this was a very handy adaptation. However, once we have reached menopause, it becomes a handicap.

protein power

Much has been made about the ability of protein to decrease blood sugar levels when added to a carbohydrate meal. The exact effect, however, depends upon both the type and amount of protein and the medical condition of the person eating the combination. In normal people (remember that's a man by scientific definition) and non-insulin dependent diabetics (NIDDM) protein stimulates insulin secretion but not glucose, which causes a drop in blood sugar. However, it requires a LOT of protein to do this. Let me give you an example: Four slices of white bread contain 50 gm of carbohydrate which act like 3 tablespoons of corn syrup in your body. It would take 50 gm of protein or 12 ounces or 3 chicken breasts to cause a drop in blood sugar in response to eating that bread.[62] If you were an insulin-dependent diabetic, you would increase rather than decrease your blood sugar levels by adding that much protein to your meal.

Women add an additional hour onto digestion

Protein, however, does stimulate the production of glucagon which, along with cholecystokinin, can help to decrease your meal size by signaling that you're full.[63] So the ability of protein to stimulate glucagon is important to those with delayed gastric emptying when protein is eaten first.

fat facts

Fat, especially saturated fat, slows down the rate at which your stomach is able to process foods. In addition, it also impedes the activity of the small bowel in propelling food along your digestive tract.[64] Delayed gastric emptying will have the effect of lowering your blood sugar response to a meal. A lot has been made about eating specific ratios of fat and protein in order to maintain normal glucose levels. This Zone approach is not in line with current research. If you put 25 gms of fat or 2 1/2 tablespoons of butter on white bread it will have no effect on preventing the sugar rise in normal people.[65] The addition of fat to a carbohydrate gives you the same blood sugar response as if you ate the carbohydrate alone but a greater insulin response. This is not good, as the longer insulin stays around, the more hostile your tissue becomes to letting go of fat. So it seems fat and protein, when added to a meal, can reduce your blood sugar response but only if relatively large amounts of either are used.[66]

Eating a breakfast full of low glycemic carbs can lower your insulin response

become a mixtress

When you eat a "mixed meal" of protein, carbohydrate and fat, the amount of blood sugar rise can be predicted from the glycemic index of the carbohydrate alone. This is significant, because only by choosing foods that are low in their ability to turn your body into a sugar cube can you achieve a more normal insulin response.[67] Furthermore, by eating a breakfast full of low glycemic carbs you can lower your insulin response to a standard lunch meal by as much as 30%.[68] An added benefit of eating low GI foods is a normal bowel movement, as nearly 20% of the undigested starch from these foods will be metabolized in the colon, acting as additional fiber in your diet.

graze or gorge

Another way to keep your blood sugar under control is to eat frequent small meals instead of one big meal. Snacking on 250 calorie "mini meals" can keep your insulin levels down, which in turn lowers your cholesterol.[60] As an added bonus, small meals relieve the stress on your body, as evidenced by lower cortisol and cholesterol levels and make it easier for your stomach to empty.[69, 70] By simply reducing the rate at which you present food to your digestive tract you can dramatically reduce the rate of lipids or fats appearing in your blood regardless of what you eat.

Are you a gorger who eats most of your calories at one meal? If you are, the saturated fat and high glycemic carbohydrates in that meal packs a whollop. You essentially overload the circuitry of your body's digestive process and cause a "blackout" which has devastating effects on your circulation, not to mention your waistline. But if you snack on 5 to 7 meals a day with the same amount of calories, you maintain an even, smooth level of sugar and fats in your blood. Your electric grid stays lit without any signs of overload. By spreading the calories of a meal throughout the course of a day your body will trigger a counter regulatory mechanism that sends growth hormone levels up for 4 hours after each meal. Remember, the more growth hormone around, the more you burn fat, not muscle.

Our bodies can tolerate a rise in fat levels between 10 to 30% and still keep the insulin, glucose and corticosterone levels low, but if we eat more than 30% fat at a single sitting we end up with elevated blood sugar levels and more fat storage.[71] By eating mini meals and spreading the calories, our bodies can handle a fat load in excess of 30% and still not lose control.[72]

can one meal affect the next?

Our bodies can be downright stingy when it comes to letting insulin out of the vault if we eat meals closer together. Known as the Staub-Traugott effect, scientists have shown the closeness of one meal to the next determines the blood sugar response to the following meal; the closer together the meals are, the better the glucose tolerance and the less insulin the body needs to keep your blood sugar in check.

The amount of fiber in a meal can also affect the burst of insulin you release when faced with the next meal. Fiber, by its sheer ability to slow down digestion, can lower blood glucose levels. High fiber soups can significantly suppress hunger and reduce the amount of calories desired in the next meal, especially if you eat a "chunky" soup.[73] But this is not the main reason the composition of one meal affects the next one's ability to raise your blood sugar. In a study of mixed meals with different fiber contents but the same glycemic carbohydrate content, researchers found that a dinner composed of low glycemic carbohydrates improved your carbohydrate tolerance for breakfast.[74] It's like having an overdraft built into your carbohydrate checkbook.

the french paradox

Now that you understand the advantages of "mini meals" you have understood a paradigm that stumped researchers for years, called The French Paradox. It seems our French relations, who helped us win our independence from England, may also be helping us lose the fat. Although the French eat a higher saturated fat diet, smoke and drink alcohol, they have 40% fewer heart attacks than Americans.

So how do they do it?

• The French are consumers of moderate amounts of alcohol, especially red wine, usually with meats

• The French eat more fresh fruit and vegetables

• The French eat less red meat

• The French consume more cheese and less whole milk

• The French use more olive oil and less butter or lard, and they take longer to eat meals and snack less on high carbohydrate foods

Now, not all things are good for all people, as you will see with wine. However, there are several important points to remember. Eating a diet high in fruit and vegetables offers your body high levels of folate, which lowers plasma homocysteine levels. Even mild to moderate elevation in blood values of this amino acid is a strong risk factor for atherosclerosis clogging up arteries to the brain, heart and limbs.[75] In a study of diet diversity and quality of the French, researchers found that few French adults consumed diets consistent with the American USDA recommendations. Only 14 % of those studied got their fat levels below 30% and less than 4% consumed less than 10% of that as saturated fat. In contrast, 90% of them had the most diverse diet, with women choosing more "vitamin dense" foods, while those who did meet the USDA requirements scored the lowest in food choices.[76,77] Much like the advice given by any financial advisor, diversity in your food choices seems to be an important factor in protecting your life's assets against fluctuations in the energy consumption market.

Although the French are not known for their

exercise clubs, their lifestyles are naturally more active. They live in small villages where they walk and their lives don't revolve around cars and malls. They shop and carry home fresh food daily and rarely prepare meals from the cupboard. Foods are available seasonally, not year round which affects the nutritional content of the food. Cars are a luxury, necessitating several episodes of walking per day with weighted packages. Meals in restaurants are expensive, so more socialization is done at wine bars or bistros where a single dish can be consumed over an hour of friendly conversation. But most of all the French understand the importance of breakfast, especially among women with low BMI or body mass index.[78] They are more aware of the importance of choosing foods that offer protection against heart disease and cancer. Eating fruits and vegetables, especially tomatoes, can protect against cancers of the digestive and respiratory tracts.[79,80] French women who are obese eat more like Americans. They don't eat breakfast, consume only three meals a day and spend more time watching television.[81,82]

The French understand the importance of breakfast

fudging with fat

Numerous studies have reported a positive link between dietary fat and fatness. However, only recently have researchers focused on the type of fat in addition to the quantity in our diets. It seems fat intake can only explain about 2% of the fat snuggled under your skin and hiding in your abdomen.[83] In a study specifically of pre and postmenopausal women, including African Americans, changes in the amount of saturated fat intake had a dramatic effect on lowering cholesterol, especially LDL or the bad low density cholesterol.[84] When another group of postmenopausal women were placed on a 26% fat diet consisting of 14% monounsaturated fats with only 6% saturated fat, they too improved their cholesterol profiles.[85] It seems fudging your fat intake by substituting more mono-unsaturated fats like olive oil can result not only in weight loss but a much better cholesterol and insulin response.[86] Even a handful of peanuts, which are rich in oleic acid can make a difference in postmenopausal women's risk for heart disease.[87]

Butter doesn't deserve the bad rep it's gotten when it comes to the effect of different fats on cholesterol levels in your blood, liver and gallbladder. While palm, coconut and olive oil caused the highest concentration of cholesterol in the blood, butter produced an intermediate response in all three categories and was not linked to gallstone formation.[88] Butter also contains buteric acid, which helps you absorb nutrients from your food. So don't be afraid to incorporate unsalted butter into your diet if you're watching your cholesterol.

digging your grave with your own teeth

Unfortunately, all these facts fly in the face of the very diet your doctor or other experts may be suggesting. The current recommended diet for women in menopause emphasizes substituting carbohydrates for saturated fat without concern for their ability to raise your blood sugar level. No wonder women are going nuts trying to figure out why they are gaining weight![89] Low fat, high carbohydrate diets increase the insulin concentration in your blood, which can raise your risk for heart disease. The more insulin resistant you become during menopause, the greater will be the negative effects on insulin, glucose and cholesterol if you consume a high carbohydrate, low fat diet. Studies bear this out.

Low fat, high carbohydrate diets increase the insulin concentration in your blood, which can raise your risk for heart disease

Two diets were tested using the following composition of carbohydrates, fat and protein: Group 1 ate a 60/25/15 ratio and Group 2 consumed a 40/45/15 diet. That's right–45% fat. The ratio of mono/poly and saturated fat were the same. As predicted, those who substituted carbs for fat had a marked decrease in the good high density cholesterol with an overall elevation in LDL /HDL ratios to above 4, which is considered dangerous.[90-92] This is not an isolated study, but rather consistent with numerous large epidemiological studies of women and their risk for heart disease.[93-96] The answer seems clear: low fat, high carbohydrate diets can cause dangerous changes in your health, especially if you are insulin resistant. It's like digging your own grave with your teeth every time you load up on high glycemic carbs. It just makes sense to decrease the saturated fat in your diet by increasing the amount of mono-unsaturated fats and low glycemic carbs instead of reaching for that potato. And if you want to maintain your weight loss during menopause, monounsaturated fatty acids are the key.[86] (Table 4)

Table 4

dietary sources of essential fatty acids

Fatty Acid	Food source	Enriched source
Linoleic acid	vegetable oils	corn oil
Alpha linolenic acid	seeds, nuts	black currant oil flaxseed
Gamma linolenic acid	seeds, nuts	primrose borage oil
Arachidonic acid	red meat	
Eicosapentaenoic acid	seafood	fish oil
Docosahexaenoic acid	seafood	fish oil

Table 5

---

diseases promoted by fat

- Coronary heart disease
- Stroke
- Stomach cancer
- Colon cancer
- Pancreatic cancer
- Prostate cancer
- Breast cancer
- Ovarian cancer
- Endometrial cancer

Trouble letting go of saturated fats? Do as I did—decrease the frequency rather than the quantity at a given meal.

fat and cancer

Everyone's blaming fats for causing cancer. Just look at the diseases listed in Table 5. While saturated fat can increase your risk, there is little evidence that monounsaturated fats affect tumors. As the American public decreased their consumption of butter and dairy, they substituted n-6-polyunsaturated oils—vegetable oils—which unfortunately have a very strong cancer promoting effect. (Table 6) As a result, there has been a direct increase in the incidence of postmenopausal breast cancer. The higher concentration of fats and phospholipids as well as increased levels of estrogen produced from the conversion of body fat to estradiol is to blame. No greater proof of the association between high dietary fat and breast cancer need be provided than to look

Table 6

oils and their composition of fats

Oil	PU	MU	Total Unsat	Sat
Olive	9	77	86	14
Canola	36	58	94	6
Peanut	34	48	82	18
Corn	62	25	87	13
Soybean	61	24	85	15
Sunflower	77	14	91	9
Safflower	77	14	91	9
Palm	10	39	49	51
Coconut	5	9	14	86

at the current rise in diseases related to dietary fats in countries like Japan and even our own 50th State Hawaii. [20,97] An intake of 40% or more of fat leads to this effect, which can be reduced by dropping the amount of saturated fat.[98]

sticks and stones

Even kidney stones seem to be caused by too much fat and carbohydrates in our diet. As Japanese diets have melded into a more Westernized format since World War II, the incidence of calcium oxalate kidney stones has increased. Oxalate, which is found in leafy green vegetables and protein, binds to calcium in urine when the saturation level goes up, due to dehydration or excess excretion of oxalate. Traditionally, stone formers have been told to avoid calcium and foods high in oxalate. But in a study done in Japan, researchers found that carbohydrate consumption and fats were the more likely culprits.[99] Calcium binds to fatty acids in the bowel, indicating that fat consumption may be closely related to oxalate excretion and stone formation. Many types of carbohydrate-rich foods contain a considerable amount of oxalate. High blood sugar increases calcium absorption from the gut in addition to creating higher levels of insulin release.[100] So what's the answer to preventing kidney stones? Eat more protein instead of high glycemic, fat laden carbohydrates.[101]

When it comes to women, the calcium you get from food can prevent kidney stones, while gulping down wads of calcium supplements increases the risk.[102] This is more likely the fault of taking supplements on an empty stomach, when oxalate levels are low, rather than an excess of calcium in the urine. If you're interested in finding more ways to prevent kidney stones, read "The Kidney Stones Handbook" by Gail Savitz and Dr. Stephen Leslie.

In another interesting twist, consuming grapefruit juice increased the risk for a kidney stone by 44%, while caffeinated coffee and wine reduced the risk.[103] Grapefruit juice alters the metabolism of many drugs, including estrogen supplements.[104] It seems this particular liquid can alter the breakdown of estrogens through natural flavonoids, making too much 17 beta-estradiol and estrone available to your tissue. So play it on the safe side and take all medication with water.

Eat more protein instead of high glycemic, fat laden carbohydrates

the protein controversy

Everyone is talking about how dangerous a high protein diet can be, blaming it for everything from osteoporosis to kidney failure. But does it really deserve such a bad rep? Dieticians warn women about too much protein in their diet based upon the recommendations of the American Dietetic Association. However, their conclusions are based upon insulin dependent diabetics and people with compromised vascular problems, especially involving the kidneys. Only recently have dieticians managed the healthy, as most of their work is done in a hospital setting where bodies are understandably under physical stress.

By eating protein you encourage your body to breakdown estrogen

When women with type 2 diabetes (non-insulin dependent) eat high protein diets, they actually decrease their blood sugar and put less stress on their kidneys than women who eat a low protein, high glycemic carbohydrate diet.[309] Worries about making your body too acid are also unfounded, as sugar and starch cause more acidosis than eating protein.[310] It seems the arginine in protein actually protects your kidneys' sensitive filtering units.[311]

Women suffering from either severe under nutrition, such as anorexia nervosa, or over nutrition have changes in estrogen synthesis and degradation. Studies have suggested that obese women produce more estrogen by using their fat as estrogen converters that simply don't turn off.[105] Anorexic women can't make enough estrogen. By eating protein, you encourage your body to breakdown estrogen quicker which protects sensitive tissue from overexposure to estrogen. A diet with 25% fat increases the ability to inactivate estrogen by further shifting the formation of benign, inactive metabolites. It makes sense that high fat diets can contribute to the development of breast and endometrial cancer because they shift the balance towards highly estrogenic, active metabolites.[106, 107]

Scientists still aren't sure how dietary protein affects osteoporosis, even though protein is an important structural component of bone. In a study designed to evaluate the relationship between hip fractures and dietary protein intake, researchers found

Table 7

---

food sources of phytoestrogens

Isoflavones	<u>Legumes</u> Soy beans, lentils, beans (haricot, broad, kidney, lima, chick peas) <u>Products of beans</u> Soy meal, soy grits, soy flour, tofu, soy milk
Lignans	<u>Whole grain cereals</u> Wheat, wheat germ, barley, hops, rye, rice, brans, oats <u>Fruit, vegetables, seeds</u> Cherries, apples, pears, stone fruits, linseed, sunflower seeds Carrots, fennel, onion, garlic Broccoli Vegetable oils including olive oil <u>Alcoholic sources</u> Beer from hops, bourbon from corn
Coumestans	<u>Bean sprouts</u> Alfalfa, soybean sprouts Fodder crops Clover

---

that eating protein, especially from animal sources, was actually beneficial in reducing the incidence of hip fractures in postmenopausal women followed for ten years.[108] Eating fruits and vegetables high in potassium also protects your bones by reversing any urinary calcium loss.[312] So don't be afraid to eat more protein. It could be just the leg you need to stand on.

friendly phytoestrogens

Phytoestrogens, which are contained in plant foods like garlic and onions, help protect against cancer by pushing the metabolism of estrogen to its less cancerous, inactive metabolites. (Table 7) Phytoestrogens are active in the body and can reduce cholesterol and help treat osteoporosis.[109,110] Garlic and onions seem to offer additional protection against breast cancer while isoflavones, found in beans and soy, had the same effect as hormone replacement therapy on relaxing blood vessels.[111,112]

The source of protein becomes important. Studies have shown protein loading with soybean meal seems to be friendlier on our kidneys than beef or chicken.[113] Some phytoestrogens, like beans and soy, are high in protein. When you enjoy a diet chock-full of these foods, you are really eating a high protein diet. So if you are concerned about consuming more protein, just make the difference up with phytoestrogens.[114] Just 40mg of isoflavones per day, the equivalent of one serving of a soy food, equals the typical Asian diet.[115] That's about 3 tablespoons of soy powder or 1.5 ounces of tofu. Just in case you thought eating lots of soy was beneficial, be aware there is a dark side to soy. Too high an intake, especially in supplements, can turn off your thyroid and interfere with your hormones, especially estrogen. It's a classic example of soy being beneficial in moderate amounts and harmful in larger amounts, just like estrogen. So use common sense. Incorporate small amounts of low-glycemic phytoestrogens into your diet along with low fat sources of protein for a healthy lifestyle.

women and alcohol

As someone who grew up in California and makes frequent trips to Napa, I can vouch for the wonderful flavor of California wines. But as a woman in menopause, I have to acknowledge wine poses a dangerous risk factor to my health. Unlike men, women who drink alcohol, regardless of the type, increase their chance of getting breast cancer by 12%, making it one of the major avoidable risk factors.[116] Since our stomachs are slower to empty, alcohol has a more intense "first pass" effect on the liver and causes even more delayed emptying.[117] We get higher blood alcohol levels with just one drink. Metabolism of estrogen is intensely affected with blood levels tripling within one hour. Drinking even raises our chances for high blood pressure and strokes.[118-120]

If, like me, you love wine, you should know that women subconsciously crave alcohol as their estrogen levels are dropping. The more we drink the higher estradiol levels can go.[121] But most of all, alcohol makes you fat by increasing your waist and waist-to-hip ratio which correlates with that hidden intra-abdominal fat.[122] In a study comparing the influence of alcohol consumption between French men and women, men had little change in their waist or weight by drinking alcohol, while a woman might as well pour a bottle through her belly button. Women are just more sensitive to the metabolic effects of alcohol and shouldn't be duped into believing the current press that wine is the way to beat heart disease, when a diet rich in fruit and vegetables can provide the same benefits.[123,124,75]

Alcohol makes you fat and raises your chance for high blood pressure and strokes

Unfortunately, little effort has been made to provide non-alcoholic wines fortified with quercitin and resveratrol, the active ingredients felt to be responsible for a healthy heart. In the United States, alcohol is the third-leading cause of premature death; its use and abuse result in more than 100,000 deaths annually and imposes more than $167 billion in economic damage on society. The rate of coronary heart disease may be relatively low, but deaths from alcohol-related digestive diseases and cancers, as well as unintentional injuries, are excessive, recently estimated at nearly 25% of all premature mortality. Official government policies in France, as in the United States, call for reductions in alcohol consumption.

Does this mean you can't enjoy the occasional

glass of Chardonnay? The operative word here is occasional. If you don't want to sabotage your shape or increase your risk for certain cancers, keep the wine for that special occasion.

caffeine : grounds for concern?

That cup of joltin' java turns out to be a lot safer than we thought in terms of cancer, but drink too much and you could sabotage your efforts to lose weight by turning off your fat burning mechanism. Dietary caffeine, specifically methylxanthine-containing beverages such as coffee and colas, have been blamed for bone loss, breast cancer and headaches. However, objective studies have been few, relying mostly on supposition and anecdotal experience. But after several studies, caffeine has been given a pardon when it comes to stealing calcium from your bones. One hundred thirty eight postmenopausal women not on estrogen therapy were measured for bone density in their hips and total body. After reviewing their caffeinated beverage use, no incriminating evidence could be found connecting bone loss with caffeine.[125] This was also confirmed in another study where researchers couldn't hang caffeine with causing hip fractures among women who drank regular or decaffeinated coffee, tea or cola.[126] Likewise, over 5000 women with biopsy proven breast cancer were followed for ten years and compared with 5000 women without cancer and no correlation could be found between consumption of caffeine and breast cancer occurrence. In fact, researchers were able to exclude caffeine as a risk factor in breast cancer.[127] And for those of you who can't live without your morning jolt of java, the risk of colon cancer was reduced in drinkers of 4 or more cups per day in over 10,000 people studied for 5 years.[128] However, a rise in blood sugar levels without stimulating insulin was found about 2 hours after drinking caffeine. So if you consume numerous cups a day, you may be turning off glucagon and your fat burning mechanism.[129]

liquid oxygen

Water is an essential but often overlooked nutrient required for life. Within your body, water is the great transporter—of nutrients, oxygen and waste products. It provides a medium for chemical reactions. It cools and cushions your body, which is composed of more than 50% water. In a way, we're a mobile aquarium in which assorted organs slosh around like buoys in an ocean. To be well hydrated the average woman needs to drink 9 cups of fluid per day in the form of nonalcoholic beverages, soups and foods. Solid food contributes about 4 cups of water with an additional 1 cup coming from the process of oxidation in the body. It's been proven that fluid consumption in general and water drinking in particular have a positive effect on the risk of kidney stone disease, breast, colon and urinary tract cancer, obesity, mitral valve prolapse and overall health.[130] Water is really liquid oxygen, made up of two parts hydrogen for every single oxygen molecule. Think of it as just another way of increasing the amount of oxygen in your body. By drinking one liter of mineral water, you can obtain nearly one half of a day's recommended dietary allowance of calcium (1000 milligrams) without any absorption problems. So next time you're reaching for a cola, try some "Liquid Oxygen" instead.

We're a mobile aquarium in which organs slosh around like buoys in an ocean

a pinch of salt

Women have blamed salt for puffy ankles, eyes and those mood changes Al Bundy swore stood for "**P**ummeling **M**en's **S**crotums"–PMS. But in reality, we need salt to balance our adrenal function. Our bodies are very complex, with the adrenals handling our steroid and salt/water balance. When you become low in salt, your blood pressure drops and you feel lightheaded. Salt attracts water into our plasma in an effort to compensate for changes in our sympathetic nervous system. While salt sensitivity is an inherited trait in African Americans, it has not been found in other races.[131] When healthy Chinese were given increasing boluses of salt over a week, up to 4250 millimoles a day (that's about 8 tablespoons), there was no change in their blood pressure response.[132] A low salt diet can actually increase your blood glucose and insulin levels, especially if you have any form of hypertension.[133] Elevated insulin levels, not sodium intake, will cause you to retain water.

the thyroid theory

Women in menopause, and especially post-menopausal women, can develop "subclinical hypo-thyroidism" detected by the presence of anti-bodies to the thyroid gland. Nearly 70% of women age 70 have subclinical hypothyroidism which is a risk factor for coronary heart disease.[134] In a study of healthy middle-aged women, 26% were found to have unsuspected subclinical hypothyroidism identified by the presence of antibodies and higher thyroid stimulating hormone levels than women without antibodies.[135] Yet treatment of this problem with thyroid is controversial and fraught with problems just from the medication alone.[136,137]

Cortisol is necessary to convert T4 into T3 by your thyroid. Women with subclinical hypo-thyroidism have elevated TSH levels (defined as greater than 2.0) and coincidentally, elevated blood insulin levels or insulin resistance. Remember that insulin will cause you to retain fluid by increasing your sensitivity to salt. Iodine was added to America's salt to prevent mental retardation from thyroid disease caused by iodine-deficient soil in areas such as the Ohio River Valley. However, iodine can cause significant changes in someone who has subclinical hypothyroidism, even in small doses.[138] In Japan seaweed wraps, which come from kelp that is high in iodine, caused marked hypothyroidism among those who ate it daily.[139] So using salt with iodine may be tipping the balance in your thyroid function causing you to puff up like a water balloon.

If you taste table salt, it has a bitter flavor due to the chemicals that are added along with the iodine. In comparison, sea salt has a sweet taste. Try switching your salt to a natural sea salt that has not been treated with additional iodine. I bet you will find it takes very little to bring a new flavor balance to your food and your weight.

sweet as sugar

Much has been made about the consumption of sugar in our country, but the intake of fructose has increased steadily in the past two decades as a more natural substitute for sugar in soft drinks and yogurt. However, fructose raises cholesterol and causes more adverse effects on collagen, creating sagging skin and brittle bones.[140] When protein and fructose without any fat or carbohydrate were eaten together, the insulin response was the same as 3 tablespoons of corn syrup. Glucagon was suppressed instead of stimulated in the presence of the combination.[141] So if you plan to eat fruit, either enjoy it one hour before a meal, add some fat or wait at least two hours after having any protein to keep your fat burning metabolism on high.

Fructose raises cholesterol and causes sagging skin

Aspartame (Nutrasweet™) and other artificial sweeteners have been studied extensively in diabetics.[142] It seems bitter tasting compounds, such as saccharin, sodium cyclamate, stevioside and acesulfame-K stimulate insulin release while sweet tasting aspartame did not.[143] Taste buds are apparently critical in signaling the pancreas to release insulin. Although I could find no studies on sea salt and iodinated salt, I suspect there is a similar response.

show me the diet!

You now have all the information necessary to understand The Menopause Diet. But before I summarize everything, I want to be sure you understand that diets don't work...only changes in lifestyle can make a change in your weight. If you don't put yourself at the top of that "TO DO" list, you will let stress and sleeplessness counteract all the good eating habits you'll develop following this program. As you can understand from all I have said in the previous chapters, the regulation of body weight is a deceptively complex process, of which food selection is just one part. Our hormones will fight to hold onto every last globule of fat if we don't gently convince them to get back in line. So how do we accomplish that?

like a trucker's mudflap

If you've ever been behind a big rig on the road, you may have been amused or offended by the figure on a trucker's mudflap. However, if you keep that image in mind, you won't forget the percentage of low glycemic proteins/fats/carbohydrates you should average in a weekly diet:

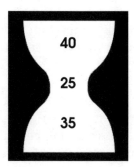

That's right. You want to select 40% of your diet as protein; keep your waistline below 30 by selecting 25% of your diet as fats and enjoy 35% of your foods as low glycemic carbohydrates; to supply your brain with enough glucose for energy. 40/25/35 – that's the plan – and the shape!

You notice I said "average" when giving these percentages. It's unrealistic to think you can manage this ratio at every meal or precisely every day. Dietary intakes vary widely, so it's reasonable to aim for a weekly average. When you eat a meal loaded with more protein, try to make your next meal a little lighter. Remember, by eating small meals frequently, you adjust your insulin response to the next meal which lets you draw or deposit into your carbo-hydrate savings account, and that spells REFUND when you consciously chose to eat a high glycemic carbohydrate or saturated fat.

How do you know if you are using the recommended "shape" of The Menopause Diet? It's very simple. Just think of your plate as a clock. Fill the portion between 12 and 5 o'clock with protein, the section between 8 and 12 o'clock with low glycemic carbohydrates and the little space left in between nicely holds a mini bowl of fat. As low glycemic carbo-hydrates contain more fiber, it's impossible to "OD" on them unlike fat, so feel free to use an extra "hour" on that clock.

how many mini meals do I need?

To lose weight, deduct one mini meal and add one half hour of exercise

It's very simple to figure out how many mini meals you need. The number of calories you burn at rest is called your basal metabolic rate or BMR. To calculate how many calories you need just to sit still, take your current weight in pounds and multiply by 11. Divide that figure by 250 and you have the number of mini meals necessary just to keep breathing. Now add 250-500 calories for walking, grocery shopping, housework or even just fidgeting and you have an idea of how many calories are required just to maintain your current weight. If you want to lose weight, simply deduct one mini meal and add one half hour of exercise a day to equal an approximate 500 calorie deficit. In just a week you will have lost one pound of fat. Keep it up and you can expect an average weight loss of five pounds the first month, and three pounds each month until you reach your desired goals.

Don't try to cheat by eliminating two meals and not exercising or eating less than 4 meals a day. You'll just lose muscle and slow down your fat burning metabolism. Then the diet fairy will come visit you and bring back all your fat plus more for good measure. That's a promise.

choosing carbohydrates

Many women prefer to know what they can't eat, rather than have a long list of all the things allowed on a diet. Since the list of "Don'ts" is rather short, and we need to save precious brain cells for remembering other things, like where we left our keys (hint...look in your other hand), I will get to the point.

don't buy

Apricots	Mango
Baked beans	Muffins
Banana	Noodles
Bread	Oat bran
Carrots	Papaya
Cereals	Parsnips
Corn	Pickles, sweet
Couscous	Potatoes
Cranberry sauce	Raisins
Dates	Rice
Figs	Yams/sweet potatoes

This also means any form of these particular carbohydrates, especially fried or buttered versions, such as potato chips or popcorn. **Remember, high glycemic carbohydrates, when treated with fat, react like 3 tablespoons of corn syrup in your body and prevent you from losing weight.** I don't mean to pronounce a sentence on all these carbohydrates and say you can NEVER eat them again, but if you want to lose the weight and feel more energized, avoid them until you have achieved the following goals:

1. A waistline below 30 inches

2. Body fat percentage below 25%

3. Body mass index below 25

In Chapter 9, I will go over how to calculate your body mass index and fat percentage. **It is not weight that determines what is healthy for each of you, but these three factors.** If you strive to achieve each one, you will have dropped your risk factors for fat related diseases down to that of a 25 year old. Now that's the true fountain of youth!

find the fat

Variety in your diet is the passbook to your weight savings account

Your gallbladder needs 10gm of saturated fat at one time in order to empty completely.[144] That is precisely one tablespoon of unsalted butter. Meats and poultry, whether red or white, have varying degrees of saturated fat. Since these are "hidden" fats, that is, you don't see the fat, it is best to restrict your intake of red meat to twice a week. I have found it easiest to restrict my saturated fat by using only 1 tablespoon of unsalted butter a day, and filling the rest of my fat allowance with mono-unsaturated fats in the form of olive oil. This has the additional advantage of cleaning up your kitchen cupboards, as you no longer need to stock every form of polyunsaturated oil. Extra virgin olive oil contains the highest amount of monounsaturated fatty acids, with the percentage dropping with each subsequent pressing of the olives. However, for salads, I prefer the less flavorful "light" olive oil. Don't confuse the name...there are no differences in calories here, only in the intensity of the flavor.

One tablespoon of butter seems skimpy unless you melt it in a very small container. Pyrex™ produces little glass containers that make a melted tablespoon look enormous. In addition, serving butter this way allows you to dip your low glycemic carbs into it, intensifying the flavor in your mouth while conserving fat grams. And don't forget to grind a few crystals of sea salt into that butter for a sweet, mouth filling flavor.

Be careful when buying foods labeled "non-fat." This does not mean low calorie as the food industry merely substitutes sugar for fat. Choose dairy products with a 2% fat content, but compare labels on any non-fat product with the full fat version to insure you're not sneaking in unwanted sugars.

If you find you just crave more saturated fat as you start the diet, try decreasing the frequency instead of the amount of saturated fat you eat in a day. Again, the French have proven variety in your diet is the passbook to your weight savings account.

protecting with protein

There are several reasons to eat more protein than currently recommended, especially in light of its ability to direct estrogen metabolism. But too much protein can stress kidneys already affected by atherosclerotic disease. The current recommendations are to consume no more than 15-20% of your diet as protein. As I have already discussed, soy protein does not cause super filtration in the kidney and provides our bodies with numerous benefits in fighting cancer and regulating cholesterol. By adding an additional 15% protein in the form of soy, you can improve your cholesterol and help protect your breast and uterine lining from any stimulation by estrogen. This is a GREAT thing!

It's easy to add soy to your diet with all the products available in today's supermarket. Try adding a tofu dog to a cup of soup, or sprinkle the powder into a hot bowl of Irish oatmeal. It's a natural for stir fry and blends up easily with Swiss Miss™ Diet Chocolate drink. Eat it as cheese or drink soy milk. The possibilities are endless. Learning to cook with soy can benefit your entire family. If you come up with a creative way to utilize soy in your diet, share it with others by posting it on my website at **http://www.menopausediet.com.** You'll find other helpful hints and "hot flash" medical information, motivational audio tapes, a newsletter, products of interest to women and a message board so you can share your struggles and success. So join in with others in making The Menopause Diet your healthy lifestyle.

fruit smoothies and energy bars

It's tempting to suggest you have a fruit smoothie for breakfast and they have become a popular way to get energy on the run. However, when protein and fructose, the natural sugar in fruit, are combined without any fat, the response in the body is the same as if you ate a piece of white bread or swallowed 3 tablespoons of corn syrup. So don't make the mistake of mixing a protein powder, such as whey or soy with water and fruit. Always make a protein drink with 2% milk. You'll keep your insulin and glucose levels under control and still have a tasty, nutritious treat. A liquid breakfast, however, doesn't balance your insulin response as well as a high fiber meal because it is absorbed at a much faster rate.[145] It's okay to use a liquid breakfast once a week, but don't make a habit of it or you'll find yourself hunting for those dangerous high sugar carbs before lunch.

When choosing fruits for your diet, concentrate on red/purple or dark blue fruits such as blueberries, blackberries, plums, huckleberries or dark red ones such as raspberries. Not only are they lower in fructose but they contain proanthocyanidins (PCA's) which can strengthen blood vessels such as capillaries and help to prevent wrinkles, varicose veins or bruising. When choosing grapefruit, red fruit contains more vitamins than pale yellow fruit with almost three times as much Vitamin A and C.

Nuts may help you lose weight and protect your heart

Energy bars are another area of potential danger. Composed of protein and carbohydrates, these bars use fructose, rice, barley or corn syrup as a sweetener and can create a "Buddha Belly" faster than you can chant a mantra! Look for new protein bars by MetRx called "Source One" which are low in fructose, sucrose and fat. As more nutrition companies focus on helping women control their glucose response, you can bet we'll see more products coming down the pipeline.

eat like an elephant

Putting away a few nuts may help you lose weight and protect your heart. Peanuts, almonds, macadamia, walnuts and cashews are excellent sources of monounsaturated fats which can keep your arteries clean as a whistle. These calorie-dense snacks are versatile and easy to incorporate into meals. Just 5 ounces is enough to provide you with 50% of your daily Vitamin E and folic acid requirements, which lowers your risk of heart disease. Nuts also contain resveratrol, the compound in red wine that prevents the oxidation of LDL in your blood. Nuts won't add inches to your waistline if eaten in small quantities but they will go a long way in helping you feel satisfied with less saturated fat in your diet. Dry roasted, unsalted peanuts are ideal for snacking and cooking. A handful is about 2 ounces, so go ahead...toss them in a salad or stew. Just don't forget to use them.

the spice in life

There is nothing more likely to evoke memories of home cooking than the smell of spices. Having traveled most of the "free inoculum world" or any-place where you don't need a vaccination, I can instantly recall a country by its smell. Cardamom, anise and cloves in Denmark to cumin, cinnamon and turmeric in Morocco—each of these combinations gets my digestive juices flowing. Herbs de Provence, a combination of french lavender, basil, thyme, savory and fennel gives all foods a new zip. As an additional benefit, fennel seeds (also known as fenugreek) help to lower blood glucose.[146] Don't forget that salt is a spice. Sometimes just a few grinds of sea salt followed by a great cracked pepper is all you need to make a gourmet dinner. Experiment with the numerous spice combinations available commercially in your market. In Appendix A of this book and on my website I will give you places to order exotic and unusual spices. With just a little variety you can make cooking as adventuresome as a trip around the world.

tea time

Tea is a medicinal drink in many cultures and a sign of friendship, as in Middle Eastern countries. Who isn't aware of the British penchant for afternoon tea or the symbolism of dumping it into Boston Harbor? Teas are really an infusion of hot water into the leaf of a plant in order to extract its essence. Some teas, such as green tea have compounds felt to protect against cancer. One cup of green or black tea has more anti-oxidant power than one-half cup of broccoli, carrots, spinach or stawberries.

With the wide variety of teas available, it's fun to make a different flavor every day. Mango and papaya teas contain enzymes that can help with your digestion of fats and proteins. It can be made by either placing a jar of cold water in the sun to process, called sun tea, leaving it out overnight, called moon tea or by infusing the mixture with hot water for 5 minutes. Look for decaffeinated teas whenever possible as they are less acidic. I enjoy Tejava, a mineral water tea made by Crystal Geyser Water Company which is available in your grocery store.

the hidden sugar : corn syrup

I was amazed when I seriously began to study food labels and discovered how many products contain corn syrup. Sold as glucose in England, corn syrup is in everything from tomato soup and juice to coffee cream substitutes. Due to the enormous excess of corn production in this country, it has become the number one sweetener in commercial products. And don't fall for rice or barley syrup as a substitute. They all have the same effect in your body. It's critical that you read the entire label on any product as you could inadvertently send your weight management program barreling off track by a simple mistake, leaving you to wonder how those fat pads hitched a ride on your hips. But here's an interesting thought—if you stick to the fresh produce section instead of the aisles of the supermarket, you won't have to be so diligent.

msg by so many names

Steering clear of monosodium glutamate, or MSG, is about as easy as dodging death or taxes. Twenty million Americans are estimated to be sensitive to this food additive which is required by the FDA to be listed whenever it is an ingredient in foods. However, there is no law requiring manu-facturers to declare *components* of any ingredient. Additives such as hydrolyzed vegetable protein (HVP), autolyzed yeast or yeast extract, and sodium and calcium caseinate all contain potentially threatening amounts of MSG, making up between 8 to 40 percent of HVP. Again, as it is used mainly as a preservative and flavor enhancing agent, that's another good reason to stay in the produce section.

portions : do they matter?

The issue of portion control is a hot one in weight management. If you're hungry, you will eat bigger portions because your brain doesn't get the signal from your stomach that it's full and had enough. Remember, hormones in your gut are responsible for emailing your brain to tell your hand to put the fork down. The greatest reason for lack of portion control is the hormonal imbalance created by delayed gastric emptying.

When I gained my weight, I was accused of having a "wooden leg" because I could eat large portions of food without feeling full. Convinced this was a misperception, I bought a kitchen scale and weighed out a single recommended portion of protein – 3 oz. It was disgustingly scrawny! I couldn't possibly exist on that little protein for my one, big meal of the day. Then I measured out a dry serving of pasta – 2 oz. My birds eat more noodles than that! Although I never tallied my calorie consumption, it was clear I was eating for more than one.

I started on The Menopause Diet without any concern for portion control and an interesting thing happened. I began cooking from the refrigerator and not the cupboard. When I started nibbling on protein first, I discovered my eyes were indeed bigger than my stomach. I stopped skipping breakfast and started to eat 5 or more meals a day. Within a week I was no longer hungry and I didn't miss the high glycemic carbohydrates I had made a staple in my diet. I was letting my body send the proper hormonal signals through cholecystokinin and glucagon to my brain. I was actually leaving food on my plate for the first time.

But things got even better. I began saving time

I cut my grocery bill in half by using the principles in The Menopause Diet and money when I shopped. By starting at the fresh produce and dairy sections, I had little need for trips down the aisles filled with shelf-stable high glycemic carbohydrates or a stop at the bakery. I experimented with the wide range of available fresh fish and selected only lean red meat for my twice weekly indulgence. The amount of food I bought dropped as I realized I could do with smaller portions of meat and more vegetables and fruit. I can now tell you, four years later, I cut my grocery bill in half by using the principles in The Menopause Diet. And who can't use more time or money?

principles of the menopause diet

Consume a diet averaging :

- 40% protein
- 25% fat (15% monounsaturated fats and 10% saturated)
- 35% low glycemic carbohydrates
- Eat 5 mini meals a day beginning with breakfast
- Exercise 30 minutes a day
- Eat 1 serving of soy a day
- Begin every meal with a mini protein starter
- Use non-iodinated sea salt
- Enjoy 5 ounces of nuts a week
- Avoid alcoholic beverages
- Drink 4 eight ounce glasses of water a day, preferably mineral water
- Reduce caffeine
- Eat low fat but not non-fat dairy products
- Use 1 tablespoon of unsalted butter daily
- Never consume fruit and proteins together without fat
- If you eat a high glycemic carbohydrate, don't add fat

chapter four
now you're cooking!

I'm bitter about Martha. You know who I'm talking about. I don't have a fabulous kitchen with color matched plates and appliances, let alone every utensil necessary to send a souffle into space. But when it comes to preparing mini meals, you don't need a designer's touch.

I'm going to share with you a sample of the many recipes I've adapted to suit The Menopause Diet. You will see that each recipe varies in its composition of protein, fat and carbohydrates, but when taken during a week, approximate the desired goal of 40/25/35. It's all just a balancing act when you're trying to lose weight, so don't be afraid to put a little "wiggle" into your diet. It's what you take in over several days that counts, not each and every bite. In a way, you could say The Menopause Diet plan is all about awareness. You make conscious decisions about the food you put into your body and you don't eat blindly.

If you enjoy the recipes in this chapter, check out "The Menopause Diet Mini Meal Cookbook." I've filled it with a cook's tour of the Mediterranean, Middle East and simply down home favorites.

allah's sunrise

This recipe comes from the Middle East and can be made as spicy as you or your family can tolerate. I enjoyed it one morning as the sun was rising over the Great Atlas Mountains in Morocco. The owner of the little store on the route to Marrakech let me watch him prepare this regional dish while his goat nibbled on the few bunches of grass outside the door.

Serves 2
per portion
Calories: 197
Protein: 9 g
Carbs: 19 g
Fat: 10 g
Sat: 2.6 g

2 teaspoons extra-virgin olive oil
1/3 cup chopped white onion
1/2 green bell pepper, seeded and cut into strips
1/2 poblano or red bell pepper,
    seeded and cut into strips
1 jalapeno pepper, raw, seeded and cut into tiny strips
    (retain the seeds and add for additional hotness)
8 ounces Muir Glen organic crushed tomatoes
    (see Resources)
2 teaspoons cayenne pepper or Aleppo pepper
    (see Resources)
sea salt
2 large eggs
Freshly ground black pepper to taste

Heat an empty cast iron skillet dry on medium heat, then add the olive oil and saute the onions and sweet peppers until soft, about 5 minutes, stirring with a wooden spoon.

Add the jalapeno and tomatoes and cook until the mixture just begins to thicken, about 8 minutes. Add the Aleppo or cayenne pepper and some sea salt to taste and adjust the seasoning for your preference.

Break one egg at a time into a bowl and slide it into the skillet while the tomato and pepper mixture is simmering. Cook for another 8 minutes, spooning the sauce over the eggs until they are set. Divide the dish in half and serve in individual bowls topped with black pepper.

classic french omelette

Serves 2
per portion
Cal: 139
Protein: 16 g
Carbs: 7 g
Fat: 5 g
Sat: 1 g

The first thing I was taught at cooking school in France was how to make an omelette. I've adapted this recipe to include soy and my favorite herbs de Provence.

1 teaspoon extra-virgin olive oil
1/2 cup zucchini, diced
2 green onions, sliced
1 large egg and 3 egg whites
3 teaspoons soy powder
1/2 cup water
1/4 teaspoon herbs de Provence (see Resources)
sea salt

In a small non-stick skillet saute the zucchini and green onions over medium heat until soft.

In a separate bowl beat the eggs and egg white with the soy powder and add enough water for consistency. Pour the mixture over the vegetables and season with salt and herbs de Provence. Split the cherry tomatoes in half and place on the left side of the omelette. When the mixture is nearly set, slide the omelette onto a plate, tipping the pan to fold the omelette in half.

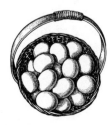

bahian black bean chili

While presenting at a conference in Rio de Janeiro, I was treated to a Brazilian dinner in the home of a friend. His wife prepared this chili which was even better the next morning for breakfast. Your family will love the samba beat it puts in your step.

Serves 8
per portion
Cal: 221
Protein: 9 g
Carbs: 38 g
Fat: 3 g
Sat: <1 g

4 teaspoons extra-virgin olive oil
1 clove garlic, minced
2 medium yellow onions, diced
1 medium poblano chili, diced
2 tablespoons cumin seed
2 tablespoons oregano
1 teaspoon cayenne pepper
1 1/2 teaspoons paprika
1 teaspoon sea salt
1/2 cup jalapeno chili, chopped with seeds
2 15-ounce cans black beans
24 ounces Muir Glen organic tomatoes, crushed
5 teaspoons soy powder
8 sprigs cilantro plus 2 tablespoons chopped
1/2 cup green onions, finely chopped
8 tablespoons white vinegar
2 medium oranges

Heat an iron skillet dry on high heat, then add the olive oil and saute the garlic, onions and poblano chili on medium heat until soft.

Add the cumin, oregano, cayenne pepper, paprika and sea salt to the mixture along with the tomatoes and chili and saute for 10 minutes on low heat.

Add the beans, soy and chopped cilantro and stir.

To serve, place the hot chili in a heated bowl, and sprinkle with some green onion. Float a tablespoon of vinegar on the top. Cut oranges into quarters and serve alongside the chili.

connemara irish oatmeal

Serves 1
per portion
Cal: 304
Protein: 20 g
Carbs: 43 g
Fat: 7 g
Sat: 2 g

My daughter and I took a trip to Ireland where we explored the countryside and frightened quite a few natives with my driving. We were served this wonderful oatmeal which I have adapted to include a portion of soy. It's better than any lucky charm!

1/3 cup Irish cut oats
1/2 cup soy milk
1 tablespoon whey protein powder
2 packets Nutrasweet™

Place milk and Irish oats in a saucepan and bring to a boil. Reduce the heat and simmer for twenty minutes until soft but still liquid. It will thicken as it stands.
Blend in the sweetener.

chilled cantaloupe and mint soup

Serves 4
per portion
Cal: 104
Protein: 4 g
Carbs: 15 g
Fat: 1 g
Sat: 0 g

This soup is wonderful in the summertime when melons are in abundance. Try using spearmint instead of peppermint for a unique flavor. If you want to get fancy, make another version with honeydew melons and pour the two into the same dish side by side for a real treat.

1 medium cantaloupe
1 1/2 tablespoons fresh mint
1 cup yogurt, low fat
1/2 cup dry white wine

Puree the cantaloupe and mint in a blender.

Pour into a bowl and mix with the yogurt and wine.

Chill overnight.

rogue river salmon omelette

Fishing on the Rogue River in Oregon is one of the simple delights in life. Chinook, Steelhead and Coho salmon run the river year round creating quite a boat traffic jam during high season. This simple omelette is a fragrant reminder of the bounties of nature.

Serves 2
per portion
Cal: 186
Protein: 20 g
Carbs: 5 g
Fat: 9 g
Sat: 3 g

1 large egg and 3 egg whites
sea salt
pepper
3 ounces smoked salmon
1 ounce goat cheese
4 small cherry tomatoes, split in half
2 tablespoons fresh parsley

Preheat oven to 350 degrees. In a small electric mixing bowl, beat egg whites with salt and pepper till stiff peaks form. In another bowl, lightly beat yolks with a fork. Fold whites into yolks.

Lightly grease an oven proof nonstick skillet and place over medium-high heat. Spread the egg mixture in the pan. Cook 3 to 5 minutes or until the bottom is lightly golden.

Place skillet in the hot oven on a medium rack and bake for 3 minutes or until nearly dry.

Dot with the goat cheese, salmon, tomatoes and parsley and bake 1 minute more. To serve, fold the omelette in half.

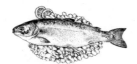

tomato and pumpkin soup

Serves 8
per portion
Cal: 110
Protein: 8 g
Carbs: 14 g
Fat: 3 g
Sat: 0 g

My grandmother was a Canadian wheat farmer's wife and she often served soup for breakfast. This unique take on a winter soup will have you in a "field of dreams" before you know it.

2 cups white onions, chopped
1 teaspoon canola oil
1/2 teaspoon nutmeg
1 can (14 1/2 oz.) pumpkin (not the one for pie)
1 can (14 1/2 oz.) Muir Glen organic tomatoes,
    chopped
1/4 cup finely chopped parsley
4 cups fat free, reduced sodium chicken stock
1 cup non fat yogurt
6 oz tofu
sea salt, pepper to taste

Heat the skillet dry on high heat, then add the oil and saute the onions on medium heat until limp and translucent.

Add nutmeg, pumpkin, tomatoes, parsley and chicken stock and simmer for 5 minutes.

Add the yogurt and tofu, puree and season to taste.

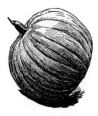

name your own vegetable soup

Asparagus is plentiful on the California coast and when it is in season I make use of every part. This soup can be turned into whatever you wish merely by using two pounds of fresh something.

2 cups fat free, reduced sodium chicken stock
3 cups water
1 pound yellow onions, chopped
3 cloves garlic, coarsely chopped
1 teaspoon extra-virgin olive oil
2 pounds fresh *something*
     (either asparagus, spinach, broccoli)
6 oz tofu
sea salt, white pepper
2 tablespoons fresh tarragon, minced

Place the stock and water into a large pot and bring to a boil.

Heat a skillet dry on high heat, then add the oil and saute the onions and garlic over medium heat until soft. Add the broccoli and season with the salt and pepper. Continue to saute the broccoli until it is bright green and starting to soften. Do not burn the onions and garlic.

Empty the vegetable mixture into the boiling stockpot and cover. Return to a boil then uncover and boil for 5 to 10 minutes, being sure not to make the broccoli lose its color.

Remove from the heat, add the tofu and puree. Add the tarragon and serve after correcting the seasoning.

Serves 8
per portion
Cal: 87
Protein: 8 g
Carbs: 10 g
Fat: 3 g
Sat: 0 g

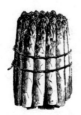

fennel and lemon soup

Serves 4
per portion
Cal: 75
Protein: 4 g
Carbs: 10 g
Fat: 2 g
Sat: 1 g

I am always looking for ways to serve unusual vegetables, and this one for fennel is easy, fast and delicious. It can be served either hot or chilled. Save some of the fennel leaves for garnish.

1 teaspoon extra-virgin olive oil
1 white onion, chopped
2 fennel bulbs, thinly sliced
2 1/2 cups chicken stock
1 cup milk 2%
sea salt, pepper
1 lemon, zested and juiced

Heat the skillet dry on high heat, then add the olive oil. Immediately reduce heat and add the onions. Cook over low heat for 5 minutes or until soft. Stir in the fennel pieces.

Add the stock and lemon zest and bring to a boil. Reduce the heat, cover and simmer for 20 minutes or until fennel is tender.

Transfer to a food processor and process until smooth. Add enough milk to give the desired consistency and season with salt and pepper. Stir in the lemon juice just before serving and garnish with some fennel leaves.

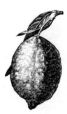

chilled chick pea, tomato and yogurt soup

Matthew Kenney of Mezze in New York serves this wonderful soup in the summer when the tomatoes are ripe and the afternoons long on sunshine. Chick peas are an ideal thickener for soup and they lose little of their nutty flavor when canned.

Serves 4
per portion
Cal: 225
Protein: 10 g
Carbs: 37 g
Fat: 5 g
Sat: 1 g

6 large, ripe tomatoes, peeled and seeded
2 teaspoons extra-virgin olive oil
2 cloves garlic, minced
1 teaspoon ground cardamom
1 teaspoon ground cumin
1 teaspoon ground ginger
2 cups canned chick peas, rinsed and drained
1 cup low fat yogurt
sea salt, pepper
12 cilantro leaves, thinly sliced

Chop the tomatoes and set aside. Put the olive oil in a 4 quart saucepan over medium heat. Add the garlic and cook for 2 minutes, stirring to avoid burning. Add the tomatoes, cardamom, cumin and ginger and cook, uncovered for 15 minutes, or until the released tomato juices start to thicken.

Transfer the tomato-spice mixture to a food processor or blender and puree. Add the chick peas, 1/2 cup at a time, pulsing after each addition. The mixture should have a coarse texture. Pour into a bowl, stir in the yogurt and season with salt and pepper to taste. Refrigerate for at least 1 1/2 hours to overnight.

To serve, divide the soup among 4 chilled bowls and sprinkle with the cilantro.

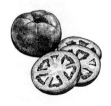

menomaise

per tablespoon
Cal: 38
Protein: 2 g
Carbs: 1 g
Fat: 3 g
Sat: 0 g

My daughter jokingly referred to my creation as menomaise when she found it in the fridge. Real mayonnaise is made with soy oil but this version works nicely as a salad dressing, dip or sauce.

1/4 cup lemon juice
1/4 cup canola oil
4 teaspoons soy sauce
1/2 teaspoon sea salt
1/4 cup yellow onions, chopped
4 green onions, finely chopped
2 cloves garlic
1/3 cup chopped parsley
1/2 teaspoon curry powder
14 ounces tofu, drained and dried

Place all the ingredients in a blender except the tofu and process.

Add the tofu and blend until smooth. Refrigerate overnight.

Makes 2 1/2 cups or 32 tablespoons

menomaise for vegetables

per tablespoon
Cal: 36
Protein: 2 g
Carbs: 1 g
Fat: 3 g
Sat: 0 g

1/4 cup lemon juice
1/4 cup canola oil
1 tablespoon dijon mustard
1 sprig fresh dill
1/2 teaspoon sea salt
14 ounces tofu, drained and dried

Place all the ingredients in a blender except the tofu and process.

Add the tofu and blend until smooth. Refrigerate overnight.

Makes 2 1/2 cups or 32 tablespoons

shrimp salad

Here's an example of menomaise at work with shrimp.

1 pound extra-large shrimp, peeled and deveined
2 tablespoons lemon juice
sea salt, white pepper
One bag of romaine lettuce or 2 large heads
6 tablespoons menomaise

Serves 4
per portion
Cal: 183
Protein: 28 g
Carbs: 5 g
Fat: 6 g
Sat: 0 g

Marinate the shrimp in the lemon juice. Season with salt and pepper, then place under the broiler or on the grill, cooking them until uniformly pink and firm, about 2 minutes per side.

Assemble the salad in individual serving bowls. Tear the lettuce into pieces and toss with the menomaise.

Add the shrimp and serve.

joel's asparagus bake

Joel is a very busy executive who finds time to cook only on the weekends. This is his easy, no holds barred approach for creating scrumptious, juicy asparagus every time. I like dipping it in my menomaise for vegetables (p.65).

Extra-virgin olive oil in a pump
1 pound asparagus, cleaned and trimmed
sea salt

Serves 2
per portion
Cal: 32
Protein: 6 g
Carbs: 3 g
Fat: <1 g
Sat fat: 0 g

Heat the oven to 400 degrees. Prepare the asparagus and place them flat in a lightly oiled glass dish. Do not bunch them up. Sprinkle with sea salt, spray with some additional oil and cover with foil.

Place in the oven on the middle rack and roast for 10 minutes. Remove the foil and roast an additional 10 minutes.

tuna and white bean salad

Serves 4
per portion
Cal: 275
Protein: 31 g
Carbs: 24 g
Fat: 7 g
Sat: 1 g

This recipe can be found in almost any Italian trattoria. It's an example of fine, clean flavors — a specialty of Mediterranean cuisine.

Dressing
3 tablespoons fresh lemon juice
1/2 teaspoon sea salt
1/4 teaspoon white pepper
1 tablespoon extra-virgin olive oil

Salad
1 pound radicchio, leaves separated
One bag romaine lettuce or 2 large heads, torn
1 red bell pepper, quartered, stemmed and seeded
1 can tuna in oil (drain the oil and reserve
    for the dressing)
1 can (15 ounces) white cannellini beans, rinsed well
2 tablespoons fresh snipped chives
2 tablespoons fresh snipped dill
2 tablespoons Italian parsley, finely chopped
2 large shallots, coarsely chopped

In a small bowl, mix the lemon juice with the salt and pepper until dissolved. Drain the can of tuna and add the oil to the olive oil. Pour the oil in a steady stream while continuously whisking the lemon juice until emulsified.

Cut the radicchio leaves into strips and toss with the torn romaine leaves. Dice the bell pepper, then add all the remaining ingredients.

Toss the salad then add the dressing to coat.

grilled chicken and mandarin orange salad

This salad is a frequent meal at my household and is so easy to make. Just serve with a glass of sparkling mineral water and Voilà!

2 cans mandarin oranges
sea salt, pepper
1 cup fresh orange juice
1/2 cup rice wine vinegar
4 boneless, skinless chicken breasts (3 ounces each)
6 cups baby spinach leaves
1/2 small red onion, thinly sliced

Serves 4
per portion
Cal: 273
Protein: 33 g
Carbs: 31 g
Fat: 4 g
Sat: 1 g

In a bowl, combine the liquid from the mandarin oranges with the fresh orange juice and vinegar. Season with salt and pepper.

Split the dressing into two bowls.

Marinate the chicken breasts in one bowl of the dressing for 15 minutes. Grill the chicken until done, about 5 minutes per side.

Toss the spinach leaves with the remaining bowl of dressing and arrange on chilled individual serving plates. Cut each chicken breast crosswise into slices and arrange them along with the oranges on top of the spinach. Strew each salad with the red onions and serve immediately.

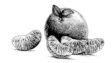

crab with spicy orange dressing

Serves 6
per portion
Cal: 138
Protein: 13 g
Carbs: 10 g
Fat: 5 g
Sat: 2 g

This dressing is excellent on shrimp, scallops or lobster and makes the fennel unusually sweet. Try using grapefruit juice instead of orange for another tasty variation. I have even served sections of grapefruit with this salad.

1 medium bulb fennel
1 tablespoon extra-virgin olive oil
3 tablespoons lemon juice
sea salt, pepper
2 cups fresh squeezed orange juice
    (grapefruit or lime)
1 teaspoon ancho chili powder (see Resources)
1 tablespoon unsalted butter
3 cans fancy white crab meat, picked for shells
1 1/2 tablespoons ground cumin
1/4 teaspoon cayenne pepper
8 basil leaves

Trim the top and bottom of the fennel bulb, then quarter lengthwise and slice the quarters into 1/8 inch slices. Place in a mixing bowl and toss with the olive oil, 2 tablespoons lemon juice and season to taste with salt and pepper.

In a small saucepan, bring the orange juice, remaining lemon juice and chili powder to a simmer over medium-high heat. Reduce to 1/3 cup, 15-17 minutes. Remove from the heat and whisk in the butter. Drain the crab and check for any shell fragments. Mix with the ground cumin and cayenne pepper.

To serve, mound the fennel strips on the plate, press down in the middle and arrange the crab meat mixture on top. Drizzle the reduced orange dressing around the base of the fennel and over the crab. Stack basil leaves and cut in julienne strips. Sprinkle on top of the crab.

moroccan orange salad

This salad was served to me in Agadir, Morocco where the evening ocean breeze is filled with the fragrance of roses. You can make this salad with either daikon (a large white radish) or fennel. One taste and your guests will be looking for your magic lamp, so make plenty.

2 small oranges
1 daikon
mint springs

Dressing:
1 tablespoon lemon juice
2 teaspoons orange-flower water (see Resources)
1 tablespoon extra-virgin olive oil
sea salt, pepper
1 tablespoon chopped mint

Peel the oranges, removing the pith and slice. Peel the daikon and slice in thin circles. Arrange the daikon and oranges in an alternating pattern on a dish.

Make the dressing by whisking together lemon juice, orange-flower water, olive oil, salt and pepper. Pour dressing over the slices and sprinkle with the chopped mint and refrigerate.

Garnish with mint sprigs and serve.

Serves 4
per portion
Cal: 70
Protein: 1 g
Carbs: 10 g
Fat: 4 g
Sat: <1 g

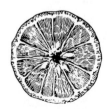

leeks nicoise

Serves 4
per portion
Cal: 109
Protein: 2 g
Carbs: 12 g
Fat: 7 g
Sat: 1 g

Here's another way to get onions into your diet. Leeks may contain dirt so be sure to split them at the bottom, make two deep cuts into the root and rinse well under water. Use a mandolin to finely slice the onions.

2 teaspoons extra-virgin olive oil
1 onion, thinly sliced
8 small leeks, cleaned
3 tomatoes, peeled and cut into eighths
1 garlic clove, crushed
1 tablespoon fresh basil, chopped
1 tablespoon fresh parsley, chopped
8 black olives, pitted and halved
sea salt, pepper
basil leaves to garnish

Heat a skillet dry on high then add the oil. Immediately reduce the heat and add the onions, cooking for 5 minutes or until soft. Add the leeks and cook, turning until just beginning to brown.

Add tomatoes. Stir in garlic, basil, parsley, olives, salt and pepper. Cover and cook over low heat 15 to 20 minutes or until leeks are tender, turning from time to time.

Remove leeks with a slotted spoon and transfer to a warm serving dish. Boil sauce for 2 minutes or until reduced and thickened. Pour over leeks and serve with basil leaves for garnish. May be presented hot or at room temperature.

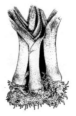

tuscany eggplant

I've never been a fan of eggplant, but this dish changed my mind. There's no need to salt the eggplant to extract any juice, so it's fast and easy to make.

2 teaspoons extra-virgin olive oil
1 onion, chopped
4 cloves garlic, minced
1 medium eggplant, peeled and chopped
2 green peppers, seeded and chopped
1 cup celery, chopped
5 Kalamata olives, chopped
1 cup mushrooms, chopped
1 can (8 ounces) tomato sauce
2 tablespoons red wine vinegar
1/4 teaspoon basil
sea salt, pepper

Serves 6
per portion
Cal: 57
Protein: 2 g
Carbs: 10 g
Fat: 2 g
Sat: <1 g

Heat skillet dry on high heat, then add the olive oil. Immediately lower the heat and saute the garlic and onion until tender. Add eggplant, green pepper and celery. Cover and cook for 15 minutes, stirring occasionally.

Add olives, mushrooms and tomato sauce, mixing thoroughly. Add vinegar and basil. Simmer uncovered until all ingredients are tender, about 15 minutes. Season with salt and pepper to taste. Serve warm.

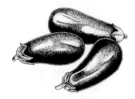

roasted sweet red peppers

Serves 4 to 6
per portion
Cal: 40
Protein: 1 g
Carbs: 4 g
Fat: 2 g
Sat: 0 g

I often make jars of roasted peppers to have on hand when I want a really great snack. They go especially well with goat cheese and basil.

4 to 6 medium red peppers
2 garlic cloves, minced
2 tablespoons red wine vinegar
2 teaspoons extra-virgin olive oil
sea salt
2 tablespoons chopped fresh basil

Roast the peppers over a flame until charred and blistered. Set in a paper bag and let cool. Remove the skins. Split the peppers in half and remove the seeds and inner membranes. Cut the peppers into wide strips.

Place in a bowl and toss with the garlic, vinegar, olive oil and salt to taste. Cover and refrigerate until ready to serve. Do not add the basil until ready to serve.

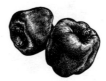

aztec zucchini

This recipe comes from Emma Gonzalez, an Aztec raised in the mountains of Oaxaca. This is one of her most requested dishes. Do not substitute the type of mint or the oil as the flavor will not be the same.

2 teaspoons peanut oil
2 cans (14 1/2 ounces) Muir Glen tomatoes
1 clove garlic, chopped
1/4 white onion, chopped
1 pound zucchini, sliced on the diagonal
1 tablespoon dried or 1/4 cup fresh spearmint,
    chopped
1/2 bunch cilantro, chopped

Heat an iron skillet dry on high heat, then add the peanut oil. Saute the tomatoes, garlic and onions until limp using a wooden spoon.

Add the zucchini, spearmint and cilantro and lower the heat. Cover and set on a low simmer for 15 minutes.

Serves 6
per portion
Cal: 95
Protein: 3 g
Carbs: 18 g
Fat: 2 g
Sat: <1 g

chili verde sauce

*Serves 12
per portion
(1/3 cup)
Cal: 23
Protein: 0 g
Carbs: 3 g
Fat: 1 g
Sat: 0 g*

Another of Emma's great sauces from Oaxaca. Watch for tomatillos in season as they are sweeter than canned. The sticky paper wrapping around them comes off easily if you rinse them under water first. If you serve this sauce over chicken, turkey or pork, just stand back and accept the applause.

1 pound green tomatillos in the husk
1 serrano chili with seeds
2 cloves of garlic
1 bunch of cilantro
1/4 white onion, chopped
1 teaspoon of cumin whole seeds
2 teaspoons peanut oil
sea salt

Steam tomatillos and chilis for twenty minutes. Cool.

Place the tomatillos, chilis, garlic, cilantro, onion and cumin in the blender on lowest setting. Once the initial chopping is done, blend on high.

Heat an iron skillet dry on high heat, then add the peanut oil and pour the mixture into the skillet. Immediately reduce the heat and simmer, uncovered until the desired consistency.

Season with sea salt.

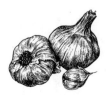

baked basque cod

Cod is a simple fish widely available in the Basque region of Spain and is a mainstay in their cooking. Try making a mixture of vegetables available in the fresh produce section for a different variation. This also works well with red snapper.

2 teaspoons extra-virgin olive oil
1 green pepper, diced
1 white onion, finely chopped
2 tomatoes, peeled and diced
1 garlic clove, crushed
2 teaspoons fresh basil
4 cod fillets, skinned, approximately 4 ounces each
Juice of 1/2 lemon
sea salt, pepper
lemon slices for garnish

Serves 4
per portion
Cal: 140
Protein: 21 g
Carbs: 6 g
Fat: 3 g
Sat: 1 g

Heat oven to 375 degrees. Brush four large squares of foil with a little oil.

Mix together the bell pepper, onion, tomatoes, garlic and basil. Put a fillet in the center of each foil piece and top with the mixture.

Drizzle with lemon juice and the remaining oil and season with salt and pepper. Fold the foil into parcels and place on a baking sheet in the oven for 20 minutes or until the fish flakes easily.

Unwrap the foil and transfer the fish, vegetables and cooking juices onto serving plates.

Garnish with lemon slices and serve.

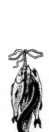

lemon tarragon chicken

Serves 4
per portion
Cal: 149
Protein: 24 g
Carbs: 0 g
Fat: 5 g
Sat: 1 g

A simple, classic French dish that takes so little time, but makes a great impression.

2 medium-size lemons
1 tablespoon chopped fresh tarragon
    or 1/2 teaspoon dried
2 teaspoons olive oil
sea salt, pepper
1 garlic clove, minced
4 small skinless, boneless chicken breasts,
    3 ounces each

From 1 lemon, grate enough peel to equal 2 teaspoons. Thinly slice half of second lemon; reserve slices for garnish. Squeeze juice from remaining 3 lemon halves into small bowl. Stir in lemon peel, tarragon, olive oil, salt, pepper, and garlic.

Toss chicken breast halves with the lemon juice mixture. Heat skillet dry over high heat.

Place chicken breast halves in hot skillet; cook 5 minutes, brushing with remaining lemon juice mixture in bowl. Turn chicken over and cook 5 minutes longer until juices run clear when thickest part of chicken breast is pierced with a knife. Garnish with lemon slices.

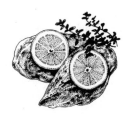

sea bass with chili and saffron

Sea bass is a popular white fish with excellent texture. It takes on new flavors when treated with this Near East recipe.

2 red bell peppers
8 Italian tomatoes, peeled*
5 tablespoons chopped cilantro
2 cloves garlic, chopped
1/2 teaspoon ground cumin
1/2 teaspoon ancho chili powder
1/4 teaspoon saffron threads
1 teaspoon paprika
sea salt, pepper
pinch of cayenne
2 teaspoons spicy olive oil
4 filets of sea bass, 4 ounces each
1/2 cup clam juice or fish stock
1 cup chick peas, rinsed and drained
harissa (optional - see Resources)

Serves 4
per portion
Cal: 261
Protein: 27 g
Carbs: 22 g
Fat: 7 g
Sat: 1 g

Char the peppers on the stove over a hot flame. If you have an electric cooktop, then preheat the broiler and put the peppers on a sheet pan lined with foil and broil for about 15 minutes, turning once or twice to ensure they blister and blacken. Place in a paper bag and let cool. Peel, seed and cut into 1/2 inch wide strips. Set aside.

Cut the tomatoes lengthwise and into eighths. Set aside.

Preheat the oven to 350 degrees.

In a small bowl, combine 2 tablespoons of the cilantro, garlic, cumin, chilis, saffron, paprika, salt, black pepper, cayenne and olive oil. If you wish a truly spicy version, add a dab of harissa. Rub each fillet with the mixture and add the remainder to the stock. Warm the stock in a small saucepan.

Place the fish tightly in a baking dish. Spread the chick peas, tomatoes, and peppers evenly on top of the fish. Pour the stock over and cover with foil. Bake for 15 minutes, remove the foil and bake 5 more minutes. Transfer the fish to a platter, surround with the vegetables and pour the cooking liquid over the fish.

Sprinkle with the remaining cilantro.

To peel tomatoes, drop them in boiling water for 30 seconds, then drop in ice water. The peel will slip right off.

indian turkey cutlets

Serves 6
per portion
Cal: 153
Protein: 28 g
Carbs: 3 g
Fat: 3 g
Sat: 1 g

This is a great way to use those turkey slices in the meat department. Be careful not to soak them in the yogurt or they will take on a mealy characteristic.

2 large limes
1/3 cup plain low-fat yogurt
2 teaspoons canola oil
2 teaspoons minced, peeled gingerroot
1 teaspoon ground cumin
1 teaspoon ground coriander
sea salt
1 garlic clove, crushed with garlic press
1 1/2 pounds turkey cutlets
cilantro sprigs for garnish

From 1 lime, grate 1 teaspoon peel and squeeze 1 tablespoon juice. Cut the remaining lime into wedges; reserve wedges for squeezing juice over cooked cutlets. In large bowl, mix lime peel, lime juice, yogurt, canola oil, gingerroot, cumin, coriander, salt, and garlic until blended.

Just before grilling, add turkey cutlets to bowl with yogurt mixture, stirring to coat cutlets.

Place turkey cutlets on grill over medium heat. Cook cutlets 5 to 7 minutes until they just lose their pink color throughout. Serve with lime wedges. Garnish with cilantro sprigs.

white bean dip with garlic, lemon and basil

This is a great dip to keep on hand for snacks. It seems I never make enough.

4 cups white beans, soaked and cooked if dried,
    or straight from can (reserve any liquid)
1/3 cup coarsely chopped fresh basil or parsley leaves
1/4 cup lemon juice
1 tablespoon extra-virgin olive oil
2 large garlic cloves, crushed

Serves 4
per portion
(1/3 cup)
Cal: 52
Protein: 3 g
Carbs: 8 g
Fat: 1 g
Sat: 0 g

Drain beans. Combine beans, basil, lemon juice, oil, and garlic in the bowl of a food processor. Process until smooth, adding reserved liquid tablespoon by tablespoon, as necessary. Add salt and pepper to taste. Refrigerate at least 1 hour.

Serve with crisp vegetables like peppers, celery, broccoli, daikon.

tuna dip

This is an updated version of an old recipe from Carlos N' Charlie's, a celebrity hangout on the Sunset Strip in Hollywood. Serve with fresh vegetables or scoop it into romaine lettuce leaves.

1 12 1/2 ounce can tuna, drained
2 jalapeno chilies, seeded and stemmed
1 (1 inch) piece green onion (green part only)
1 (1 inch) piece celery
1/4 cup light mayonnaise
sea salt, pepper
4 leaves cilantro, chopped

Serves 10
per portion
(3 tablespoons)
Cal: 69
Protein: 10 g
Carbs: 0 g
Fat: 3 g
Sat: 1 g

Blend tuna, jalapenos, green onion and celery in a food processor or blender (do not puree). Blend in mayonnaise and seasoning. Blend to desired consistency and sprinkle with cilantro.

These are recipes for seasonings that can make any simple dish a gourmet delight. I keep them on hand for grilling and they really bring out the flavor of poultry when placed under the skin.

tunisian seasoning

1 teaspoon sea salt
1/4 teaspoon cumin seeds
1/4 teaspoon corriander seeds
1/4 teaspoon fennel seeds
1/4 teaspoon Allepo pepper (see Resources)
1/8 teaspoon nigella (see Resources)

Place in a spice grinder and blend. Store in an airtight container.

moroccan seasoning

1 tablespoon paprika
1 teaspoon turmeric
1/2 teaspoon cumin
1/2 teaspoon cinnamon
1/2 teaspoon ginger

Blend and use with any liquid to baste fish or poultry.

california bbq seasoning

I have used this seasoning combination on ribs and chicken with no complaints from any of my guests. I often place it under the skin of a turkey or chicken for extra flavor.

1 cup of kosher salt
1/2 cup garlic powder
3 tablespoons cayenne
1 tablespoon white pepper
1 tablespoon black pepper
1 teaspoon onion powder

ras el hanout

This is the "top of the shop" spice mixture from Morocco. In its classic form it has 27 spices, but here is a much simpler version. You can also obtain various mixtures by direct mail. (see Resources)

1 teaspoon cumin seeds
1 teaspoon ginger
1 1/2 teaspoons coriander seeds
1 1/2 teaspoons black peppercorns
    (preferably tellicherry)
1/4 teaspoon cayenne pepper
4 whole cloves
6 allspice berries
1 1/2 teaspoons ground cinnamon
    (preferably Mexican)

Grind in a spice mill and store in an airtight jar.

italian seasoning

I first enjoyed this seasoning at Tra Vigne restaurant in Napa Valley. It was served on their grilled roast chicken. You will never eat plain chicken again after tasting this.

1 cup sea salt or kosher salt
3 tablespoons pasilla chili powder (see Resources)
2 tablespoons Ancho chili powder (see Resources)
1 tablespoon fennel
1 tablespoon cumin
1 teaspoon coriander

Grind in spice mill and store in a covered container.

fourth of july cottage cheese

Serves 1
per portion
Cal: 227
Protein: 32 g
Carbs: 20 g
Fat: 5 g
Sat: 3 g

There is nothing faster than cottage cheese and fruit when you need to get out the door in a hurry. Berries lend a festive reminder of this holiday celebration, but don't substitute nonfat cottage cheese, as the fructose in the fruit will act like 3 tablespoons of corn syrup in your body.

1 cup 2% cottage cheese
1/4 cup blueberries
1/4 cup raspberries
1/4 cup strawberries

apple in dutch chocolate

Serves 1
per portion
Cal: 101
Protein: 2 g
Carbs: 25 g
Fat: <1 g
Sat: 0 g

Gillian Anderson gave this secret away. Any fruit will do, but Fuji or Gala apples seem the tastiest when dipped in this chocolate powder.

1 Fuji or Gala apple
1 package Swiss Miss™ Diet Hot Cocoa Mix

Cut apple into wedges. Do not peel.
Rip package of hot cocoa mix open. Hold in your non-dominant hand.
Carefully dip the apple wedges into the mix and enjoy!

yogurt and nuts

Serves 1
per portion
Cal: 161
Protein: 13 g
Carbs: 17 g
Fat: 5 g
Sat: 2 g

This is another quick, easy snack to use.

1 cup low-fat yogurt
1 teaspoon slivered almonds

fruit with string cheese

I keep small individual packages of string cheese to eat with any fruit.

1 package string cheese
1 pear

Serves 1
per portion
Cal: 178
Protein: 8 g
Carbs: 25 g
Fat: 7 g
Sat: 0 g

tofu and veggies snack

2 ounces firm tofu
1/3 teaspoon olive oil
1/2 package dry onion soup mix

Place in blender until smooth. Refrigerate. Use with crisp vegetables for dipping.

Serves 1
per portion
Cal: 113
Protein: 10 g
Carbs: 4 g
Fat: 7 g
Sat: 0 g

kir royale mold

2 cups boiling water
1 package (8 serving size) JELL-O brand Sparkling
　　White Grape sugar free low calorie gelatin dessert
1 1/2 cups club soda or mineral water
2 tablespoons creme de cassis liqueur
1 tablespoon whipping cream
2 cups raspberries

Serves 8
per portion
Cal: 38
Protein: 2 g
Carbs: 4 g
Fat: 2 g
Sat: 1 g

Stir the boiling water into the gelatin in a large bowl at least 2 minutes until completely dissolved. Refrigerate 15 minutes.

Gently stir in the cold club soda, liqueur and whipping cream. Refrigerate for 30 minutes or until slightly thickened (the consistency of unbeaten egg whites). Gently stir for 15 seconds and add the raspberries.

Pour into a 6 cup mold and refrigerate for 4 hours or until firm. Unmold and garnish as desired.

white sangria splash

Serves 8
per portion
Cal: 82
Protein: 3 g
Carbs: 8 g
Fat: 2 g
Sat: 1 g

This recipe comes from the JELL-O people and makes a sophisticated dessert that's low in calories yet packed with fruit. If you use mineral water you can get your calcium too!

1 cup dry white wine
1 package (8 serving size) JELL-O brand lemon flavor
      sugar free low calorie gelatin dessert
3 cups cold club soda or mineral water
1 tablespoon lime juice
1 tablespoon orange juice
1 cup green and/or red grapes
1 cup sliced strawberries
1 cup yogurt
2 tablespoons whipping cream

Bring the wine to boil in a small saucepan. Stir boiling wine into gelatin in a medium bowl at least 2 minutes until completely dissolved. Stir in the club soda, lime juice and orange juice. Reserve one cup of the gelatin at room temperature.

Place the bowl of gelatin in a larger bowl of ice water. Let stand about 10 minutes or until thickened, stirring occasionally. If the spoon drawn through the mixture leaves definite impressions, it is ready for the next step.

Add the grapes and strawberries. Pour into three 2 cup molds or one 6 cup mold. Refrigerate about 2 hours or until set but not firm (should stick to your finger).

Stir the yogurt and whipping cream into the reserved gelatin with a wire whisk until smooth. Pour over the gelatin mold.

Refrigerate 4 hours or until firm. Unmold. Garnish as desired.

spicy fruit salad

1 16-ounce can sliced peaches
2 3-inch-long cinnamon sticks
  (use Mexican cinnamon if available)
3/4 teaspoon ground allspice
2 large navel oranges
2 large pink grapefruits
1 small pineapple
2 pints strawberries
3 kiwifruits
2 tablespoons chopped crystallized ginger

Serves 8
per portion
Cal: 106
Protein: 2 g
Carbs: 26 g
Fat: 1 g
Sat: 0 g

Drain syrup from peaches into small saucepan. Place peaches in large bowl.

Over medium-high heat, heat syrup, cinnamon, and ground allspice to boiling. Reduce heat to low; cover and simmer 10 minutes. Set syrup mixture aside to cool while preparing fruit.

Grate peel from 1 orange; set aside. Cut peel from oranges and grapefruits.

To catch juice, hold fruit over bowl with peaches and cut sections from oranges and grapefruits between membranes; drop sections into bowl.

Cut peel and core from pineapple; cut fruit into 1 1/2-inch chunks. Add pineapple to fruit in bowl.

Pour syrup mixture over fruit in bowl. Add grated orange peel; toss. Cover and refrigerate until ready to serve.

Just before serving, hull strawberries; cut strawberries in half if large. Cut peel from kiwifruits. Slice each kiwifruit lengthwise into 6 wedges. Toss strawberries and kiwifruits with fruit mixture. Place fruit salad in serving bowl. Sprinkle with crystallized ginger.

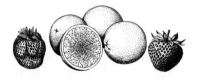

roasted peaches with cardamom

Serves 6
per portion
Cal: 78
Protein: 1 g
Carbs: 11 g
Fat: 4 g
Sat: 1 g

I never knew that roasting peaches could taste so good. Just inhale the fragrance as you serve them and you'll think you're lost in an orchard in Georgia.

6 ripe, firm peaches
1 tablespoon lemon juice
1 tablespoon unsalted butter
1 cinnamon stick, broken into 3 pieces
pinch of ground cloves
1 tablespoon ground cardamom
1 tablespoon grated lemon zest
3 tablespoons almond slices
1 small bunch mint leaves

Preheat oven to 400 degrees.

Dip the peaches in a pot of boiling water for 30 seconds, then place in ice water. Remove from the water and peel the skin. Quarter the peaches, removing the pits. Gently rub with lemon juice to prevent discoloration.

Melt the butter in large saucepan and add the cinnamon, cloves, cardamom and lemon zest. Cook over low heat for about 15 minutes, stirring occasionally. Add the peaches to the spicy butter, toss gently and transfer to a roasting pan. Bake for 15 minutes.

Arrange on a platter, sprinkle almonds and mint on top of the fruit.

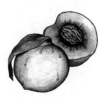

strawberries with cassis, balsamic vinegar and mint

This is an ingenious Italian dessert that presents a rich sweet and sour taste. I first enjoyed this at the La Varenne Coking School in Paris.

1 pound strawberries
2 tablespoons creme de cassis
1 tablespoon balsamic vinegar
6 large mint leaves, cut into slices
black pepper

Cut the berries in half.

Toss with the creme de cassis and refrigerate, covered for one hour or more.

Just before serving, toss with the balsamic vinegar and mint. Crack fresh pepper over top.

Serves 4
per portion
Cal: 92
Protein: 1 g
Carbs: 16 g
Fat: 1 g
Sat: 0 g

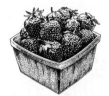

chapter five

*investing in your
health with exercise*

I'll admit right now I'm not an exercise expert. I
don't like to sweat, and I'm really not good at it! Even
mentioning the "E" word can make me break out in
a rash. I've been known to turn bright red, feel like a
furnace and get a heart rate that rivals the hammering
of a fire alarm just passing a gym. Let's face it - I
belong to the school of thought that if God had
wanted women to exercise, He would have strewn the
floor with diamonds.

Only about 38% of women over the age of 19
exercise regularly, and only half of middle-aged
women engage in any regular recreational exercise.[147,148] The benefits of exercise are well known: it
improves circulation, strengthens bones, lowers
blood pressure, cholesterol and can be key in
controlling your weight. So why are less than 25% of
women following the National Institutes of Health's
recommended guidelines for light to moderate
exercise for at least 30 minutes a day, 6 days a week?

I'll be up front with you. I HATE EXER-
CISING, but I've come to realize it is a necessary evil
in life, like mammograms. I get no high when I work
out or feel that rush of *something* that's supposed to
make you feel great. Never did, even when I danced.
Instead exercising is all work, not pleasure for me and
that's a problem in keeping me motivated. In
addition, many forms of exercise aren't really safe or
suitable for those of us who enter menopause as exercise virgins. I have a graveyard of exercise products
buried under my bed that promised to tone and

condition my body in just a few minutes a day. But then, you're talking to a woman who still believes the weight on her drivers license is valid. So what made me change my mind?

The more you exercise, especially if you participate in intensive physical activity, the stronger your bones and the less belly fat you retain in menopause.[149,150] Exercise counteracts the decline in our ability to burn fat as a menopausal mamma.[151] When you vigorously exercise, such as running or playing several games of tennis, you can significantly lower the amount of dangerous intra-abdominal fat you carry.[152,153] But here's the catch - women who are overweight are the least likely to exercise vigorously, and even moderate physical activity has little or no effect on weight control or cholesterol levels in women.[154]

Say what?? The facts are clear: **men, unlike women can raise the good cholesterol (HDL) and lose that Buddha Belly simply by dieting, while women require vigorous exercise in addition to calorie restriction to produce the same effects.**[21] Men simply have more muscle mass, which translates into a higher resting metabolic rate.[155] To make matters worse, it doesn't make any difference if a man just barely exercises. He gets the same health benefits regardless of the degree of intensity. Not so for women.[156]

The gods must be having a good laugh at menopausal women because how else could you explain this cruel inequity? I searched diligently for contradicting evidence, any scrap of research that could prove women can lose and maintain weight loss without exercise - and that is when I experienced my own epiphany about exercising. Like "red shirting" in college, I had been given a pass in the exercise game during my premenopausal years. Shamelessly, I stood on the sidelines cheering all those other women who, like me, broke a sweat just getting their nails done. But now it was payback time

The more you exercise, especially if you participate in intensive physical activity, the stronger your bones and the less belly fat you retain in menopause

and I was determined to start winning the game of weight control.

I started out by picking up fitness magazines and reading how other people conquered their aversions to exercise. Then I made a list of all the reasons I wanted to be healthy for the next twenty five years and hung it on the fridge. I itemized all the things I hated about exercise then listed ways to compensate for each one. It turned out I really had only a few objections to the Big E - sweating, boredom and pain. Then I looked at my exercise options.

run larrian run

A patient once told me she was fine until one day she ran BAM, right into menopause. I know how she feels. I have never been a fan of running. I don't see the point. Anthropologically, why would you run for hours, like in a marathon? Running is for catching something, maybe food or fleeing danger. Our pelvis, unlike a man's, was not built to withstand the bouncing tension on the pelvic floor which can lead to nerve damage. Sure the outfits are cute but I don't look good in a sweatband. Since running long distance may or may not prevent estrogen-deficient bone loss in dieting postmenopausal women, why do it?[157,158]

Aerobic exercise, which is any kind of sustained low intensity activity like walking, swimming, jogging or rope jumping, lowers your insulin response and helps to keep your blood sugar in line.[159] While some women find running a form of meditation in motion and feel their best if they run, I found it boring and painful. Besides, I wanted not only to improve my stamina but get a great shape. However, I passed on running for another reason and that was the risk of injury occurring to my knees.[160]

The normal anterior cruciate ligament (ACL) is critical for keeping your knee joint stable and aligned. Rupture of this ligament can be devastating as your knee becomes like a rocking horse with any motion, further injuring the meniscus, or gel pad in the joint which can lead to arthritis. Injuries to the ACL are four to eight times higher in women than men, especially during ovulation.[161] Estrogen, particularly the natural form of ERT, 17 beta-estradiol, reduces collagen synthesis and weakens the ligament, making it more susceptible to injury.[162] Since women live longer than men but spend more years disabled, I wanted to avoid any method of exercise that ran an increased risk of injury. This is not to take anything away from women who *enjoy* running. Remember, the key to sticking with any program is making it less work and more play. Do a risk/benefit analysis. Just be sure the **enjoyment and benefits** you receive from any exercise option are more than the relative risk of injury.

Treadmilling seemed a more logical way to avoid the chance of injury and still improve my cardio-vascular system. A word of advice: don't purchase a unit with a motor rated less than 2 horsepower or the belt won't move smoothly and you can increase your risk of injury. Always start out with a slow warmup and then hit your stride. "Milling" is a much better weight-bearing exercise for preventing osteoporosis than a stationary bike. Besides, you can't skip on a bike.

No room for a treadmill? Purchase a beaded jump rope. This type of rope is a little more weighted and balanced than a cloth, nylon or leather rope. To choose the right size, just stand with one foot on the middle of the rope and the ends of the handles should reach and barely touch your armpits. In just a few minutes of jumping in place, you can turn on your fat burning metabolism, build bones and improve your coordination.

bent on riding

I don't like riding a bike. In fact, you could say I am "biking impaired" when it comes to handling anything with two wheels. But that all changed when

I tried a "bent" or recumbent bike. It's the most fun I've ever had in a horizontal position. Okay, so I'm lying. With an estimated 15,000 recumbents sold in 1998 alone, these bikes are becoming a serious mainstream alternative for women who want a comfortable, knee-safe mode of transportation. Because you pedal in a recumbent position, it's ideal for people with short little arms and legs. Think of it as taking a spin on a Barcalounger but without the dorky looks.

What makes the ride so great? The special cantilevered fork on the load-bearing rear wheel acts as a shock absorber and the seat cushion is padded with a great back support. You can pedal longer without tiring, which helps you to burn more fat. Your butt will shape up too because bents do less for your quads and more for your hamstrings and glutes. As for other body parts, cycling in the recumbent position lets you bear less weight on your wrists, knees, shoulders and neck.

If you're like me, crashing can be a hazard to one's health. The good news? You run into objects feet first. It only took me ten minutes to learn how to ride the new BikeE CT, now christened The Hot Flash, making it the hands-down winner for biking virgins. Oh, and did I mention it's really a hunk magnet? Oh yeah! With a shape like a low rider, men will be begging you to let them try it. Just ignore the whimpering.

resisting change

It's the most fun I've ever had in a horizontal position

Working with weights or resistance training overcame many of my objections to exercise. I didn't have to sweat to get the benefits of stronger bones and muscles; it wasn't really painful and it was only moderately boring. But there are different ways to achieve resistance and with them come differences in the shape your body develops.

Lifting weights has been the standard of resistance training. You can see the results from strength training in less than three months.[163,164] A word of caution: It's safest to start with a trainer in order to prevent injury. Don't use heavy weights unless you want to look like Arnold! Instead, very light weights and a high number of repetitions will give you the tiny biceps that can lift groceries or grandchildren. If you are looking for flexibility, weights are not the answer as they tighten your muscles, instead of stretch them.

pilates®

This form of resistance training has seen a new resurgence as women are looking for a long, lean look to their bodies. Developed as a rehabilitation program for injured soldiers during World War I, Pilates® emphasizes flexibility along with strength. When combined with controlled breathing, it offers a great workout. By isolating certain muscle groups, no unnecessary energy is expended and weak muscles are strengthened as bulky muscles become elongated. It's really a form of "dancing on your back" with smooth gliding motions.

The secret to Pilates® is learning posture and how to keep your abdominals taut while moving your arms and legs. It requires mental focus, as these exercises engage the whole body and mind, challenging you to concentrate on body alignment and control. It's truly a way of bringing conciousness to your muscles.

I have faithfully done this exercise program for a year, which tells you it is neither boring, sweaty nor painful. However, it is expensive and requires special equipment. You really need to do it with an instructor if you want to achieve the full benefit of this program. Pilates® is not a replacement for cardio conditioning as it is really anaerobic exercising. There are floor exercises which you can follow from several books.

yoga

Yoga offers much of the same benefits as Pilates® without requiring any equipment. There are four key exercises that will teach you the ABC's of yoga. The first one is called the Mountain pose. You literally stand like a mountain, stretching your fingers downward while feeling like a string has been drawn through the top of your head, pulling your spine upwards. This positions raises awareness of how you stand and improves your posture. The second position is the Tree pose. I think of it as standing like a stork on one foot with your other foot planted firmly against your thigh while raising your arms above your head. Balance is the key here. Just don't try this one when your dog decides to run laps around the room. The third position involves sitting on the floor with your legs and toes extended while drawing in your abdomen. This is a quiet, meditative type of position. Finally, you can sit on your heels while breathing in slowly for 2 to 3 minutes in order to connect and center yourself.

The deep breathing of yoga, combined with its stretching, is an excellent way to begin any exercise plan. The goal of exercising is to increase the exchange of oxygen by every cell in your body. Certain forms of yoga emphasize breathing in specific patterns, which can be helpful in managing hot flashes. There are numerous videos and books on this technique which can help to limber you up for that position on page 28 of the Kama Sutra.

endurance is the key

If your goal is to firm, tone or reduce, you want to concentrate on developing good muscle endurance. That means you can hit a golf ball 200 yards on the first hole and 200 yards on the eighteenth hole four hours later. Low glycemic index carbs can do the trick because they result in higher concentrations of fuels towards the end of your exercise program when you need them most.[165] So don't rush to eat that high sugar energy bar before playing tennis. You'll only be giving your opponent the advantage. Munch on some broccoli or cottage cheese instead and stay cool to the finish.

the secret to my success

You can do anything for ten minutes

I really wish I could tell you I went to bed and woke up refreshed and ten pounds thinner, but that would only be "in my dreams." I selected a program of cross training using Pilates® two days a week, biking on my recumbent and walking on a treadmill twice a week which I conveniently placed under a ceiling fan and smack dab in front of a TV with a remote control. In this way I could stay cool and stave off boredom by watching my favorite movies or comedy shows.

You can lose weight and fat without compromising your muscle strength if you do strength training three days a week and walk two more days.[166] If you only use The Menopause Diet, you'll miss the opportunity to increase your muscle mass and its ability to burn fat.[167] In short, you'll be flying on low octane instead of jet fuel. Don't have enough time to exercise? Even short bursts of brief intense exercise can lower your sugar and insulin levels.[168] Try breaking your exercise into 10 minute segments. Come on...you can do *anything* for ten minutes! Take the stairs, walk to the book store or just around the block. Seize the moment and get on the treadmill while watching the news. Flexibility is the key to making exercise work for you. Treat each day like a menu - mix and match and you get a full course. As I stated, I am no exercise expert, but you will find lots of resources to explore in Appendix A to help you find an exercise program that works for you.

High blood pressure is a killer but regular moderate exercise, such as walking, can significantly lower your risk of a stroke.[169] It can also nudge a sluggish gallbladder into action.[170] So don't just choose one type of exercise - mix it up and your body will thank you. And remember all those ballet and gymnastic classes your mom forced you to take? Exercising during puberty is an opportune time to increase bone density that can last into your "Golden Years" by reducing the risk of fractures after menopause.[171] This only proves mothers really DO know what's best!

Estrogen, when combined with The Menopause Diet and treadmilling, can give you the same benefits as intensive exercise because the combination enhances your ability to send growth hormone levels shooting up. Now you can really burn the fat hiding deep inside your stomach.[172,173] Even strength training results in stronger bones with the assistance of estrogen.[174] Again, micro managing your hormones is important, as I will discuss in the next chapter, so work with your physician to modify your dosage to suit the lowest level possible that will still give you heart, brain and bone protection.

After just three months of following The Menopause Diet Plan of mini meals and exercising, I had lost enough weight and inches to stand in the far corner of my closet looking at clothes I hadn't worn in 10 years. Suddenly, sleeves were waving furiously at me and I swore I heard cries of "Pick Me... Pick Me...I haven't been out in years! Who looks best on you baby?" But then again, maybe it was the hot sauce talking.

chapter six

are hormones
making you fat?

At a party in Beverly Hills, a woman ran into an old friend who looked beautiful and radiant. "She's just my age," said the lady, whom I knew to be 51. Then she whispered in my ear "I bet she's on estrogen. Women in this town will do anything to look young, even if it means getting cancer." Whether to take hormone therapy is a decision every woman ultimately faces. With over 21 million women of the baby boom generation entering menopause this decade, small wonder hormone therapy has replaced sex, kids, jobs and cooking as the number one topic of conversation among middle-aged women. This was dramatically brought home to me at an after-dinner gathering in which the husband of one of my friends stood up amongst the women and said "I know where this conversation is going...where it's always going....." pointing 'down there' as he left the room. And he was right!

the weight connection

It's a myth that estrogen causes weight gain. Unfortunately, physicians mistake the changes that come naturally with menopause and aging as due to estrogen therapy. Nothing could be farther from the truth.

The Rancho Bernardo study examined whether long-term postmenopausal hormone replacement therapy (HRT) was linked to measures of obesity and found that HRT, when used either intermittently or continuously for 15 years or more was NOT associated with the weight gain and intra-abdominal fat commonly seen in women.[175] In fact, women who use hormones have a significantly trimmer body than women who had never used HRT.[176,177] This makes sense when you remember that growth hormone and estrogen help to mobilize and burn fat. Excess weight, central obesity, diet changes and lack of exercise are more to blame on advancing age, which leads to altered glucose tolerance and increased insulin resistance.[39] Estrogen deficiency is responsible for failing to stimulate the pancreas to secrete insulin. The great news – this can be reversed by estrogen treatment **IN SMALL DOSES!** By contrast progestins, the synthetic androgens, counteract these effects of estrogen and may actually promote insulin resistance and hyperinsulinism. This is a very bad thing!

the fat lady at the circus

A cluster of changes occur when women have more male hormone or testosterone production. As estrogen and progesterone levels drop, the adrenals put out large amounts of steroids such as dehydroepiandrosterone-sulfate (DHEA-S) and androstenedione, which are changed into androgens or estrogens by fat tissue. In fact, the conversion of these steroids by fat into estrone, a poor relation of estrogen, is the only source of estrogen in post-menopausal women not on HRT.[178]

A lack of estrogen can also make you look manly, develop facial hair and even go bald. The fat lady at the circus with the mustache is no accident. You can even develop acne, like a teenager, but without the sex drive to compensate. Women with too much testosterone actually have a higher rate of heart disease.[179]

Menopausal women who don't take estrogen thicken their hearts, which makes it more difficult to pump oxygenated blood throughout the body. Once this happens, your blood pressure goes up.[180,182] The good news? Just taking estrogen brings everything under control.[183]

the horn of plenty

Never before has so much information about the benefits of estrogen been reported in scientific journals, yet only one in three women over 50 is on hormones. At issue is whether menopause is seen as a "disease" that requires medical intervention or a natural aging process that should run its course without treatment. In 1997, the Gallup Organization conducted a poll of women 45-60 years of age regarding their sources of information on menopause, what changes in health they anticipated as a result of menopause, why they used hormone therapy and their attitudes toward menopause as a natural or medical event. The results were disturbing. Women were more likely to believe that depression, hot flashes and irritability were associated with menopause than heart disease, vulnerability to Alzheimers, osteoporosis or stroke.[184]

In another study, the most frequently cited reasons for taking hormones are menopausal symptoms, osteoporosis prevention and physician advice.[185] In Great Britain, many women make decisions about HRT independent of their interactions with health care providers, relying upon friends, relatives and the media as important sources of information.[186] Our Australian sisters fare little better, with nearly 40% of women currently using HRT, mainly due to hysterectomies.[187] Whether or not a woman uses HRT is dependent upon the perception of her menopausal status, excessive fear of breast cancer, the belief that hormones are unnecessary because menopause is a natural event or not wanting menstrual periods.[185-188]

European women fluctuate widely in their use of HRT with only 13% of post-menopausal women choosing therapy. About half of the women admit never discussing menopause or its symptoms with their doctors, yet two-thirds of the women studied believe they needed more information about HRT.[189] Again, the most common reason given for stopping therapy was having a period.[190]

it's all a misunderstanding

A lack of understanding of the long-term consequences of menopause seems to be a major contributing factor to the low demand for hormone replacement. While 96% of women can define the menopause, there is an appalling lack of awareness of the problems of either osteoporosis or cardiovascular disease in post-menopausal women and only 8% of women know that HRT can be used to treat them.[191] African-American and British women are often treated incorrectly, while those in whom the greatest benefit could be derived — women with diabetes and cardiac disease — are not offered HRT.[192-194]

coast to coast

So what predicts a woman's use of hormone replacement therapy? Women who are white, have undergone a hysterectomy, are more highly educated or live in the West have a higher rate of hormone usage.[195] But there is a particular group of women who are nearly twice as likely to use HRT - and that is women doctors.[196,197] In a study conducted by Emory University in Atlanta, women doctors are more likely to use HRT "because they have a greater ability to scientifically evaluate the benefits and risks" says Dr. Sally McNagny, author of the study. I was personally amused when the breakdown of HRT users ranged from 8% in Massachusetts to more than 40% on the West Coast with a national average of 24%. Not

Women doctors use HRT because they can scientifically evaluate the benefits and risks

surprisingly, they are significantly more likely to be gynecologists with 60% of women physicians between 40 and 49 using HRT compared with 49% between the ages of 50 and 59 and 36% of those 60 to 70 years old. Women physicians have a few other notable traits: they are much more likely not to smoke or drink alcohol. In fact, the reported behaviors of women physicians exceed national goals for the year 2000 in all examined behaviors and screening habits for a healthy lifestyle.[198] Our British compatriots are no slouches either. Women doctors in England use HRT to prevent osteoporosis and heart disease in 73% of those surveyed, while selecting a lifestyle that includes skim milk, a lot of fruit, vegetables and fiber, along with vigorous physical activity at least once a week.[197] It seems women doctors are voting with their prescription pads to support HRT with long term prevention in mind.

a call to action

One third of women between the ages of 45 and 75 have cardiovascular disease, which accounts for more than **34% of all deaths among women annually**.[199] Nearly 367,555 women die from heart disease compared to 20,200 from breast cancer and 27,500 from lung cancer. Women who experience a heart attack are older and suffer more often from diabetes, hypertension or previous angina and develop more severe infarctions than men.[200] Premenopausal African American women have more risk factors than white women with a greater body mass index and a much higher consumption of saturated fat and cholesterol.[201] The statistics tell a very different story from women's perceptions that heart disease is a "man's disease" and that women are protected until menopause.

unraveling the tangled web

A substantial body of evidence shows that HRT protects women against cardiovascular disease.[202] Estrogen has a significant dose-dependent response in its ability to cause blood vessels to relax when faced with a clot. Estrogens possess anti-atherosclerotic properties at low concentrations while clogging arteries at high concentrations, a classic example of " if a little bit is good, a whole lot is NOT better."[203,204] When it comes to insulin resistance, which can lead to diabetes, 50% of young women have some degree of abnormality in the breakdown of carbohydrates and the severity of this effect increases after menopause. Insulin sensitivity and glucose tolerance are improved by the use of natural estrogens such as estradiol, which is derived from plant sources.[21]

Women who use estrogen have a much lower risk of tooth loss

Estrogen users, in contrast to non-estrogen users are able to reduce their risk of coronary heart disease by 44% and are less likely to have coronary artery stenosis.[205] The benefits of estrogen seem to be the same regardless of your ethnic makeup. The Strong Heart study of American Indian women found that estrogen users have a significantly lower level of the bad cholesterol (LDL) and fibrinogen, which contributes to clot formation, and higher values of the good cholesterol (HDL) while maintaining a slim figure.[206]

them bones, them bones

But there may be another good reason to consider estrogen therapy. Estrogen has been shown to dramatically reduce bone resorption and increase bone formation.[207] Osteoarthritis is higher in women than men, and your chances of developing it increase dramatically in the years after menopause.[208] It seems women are prone to a particular hand osteoarthritis affecting the thumb due to cartilage's sensitivity to estrogen. In the absence of estrogen, the body produces increased levels of killer white cells that attack collagen sites, including your gums.[209] Women who use estrogen have a much lower risk of tooth loss, which is good news if you're haunted by the sight of a pair of choppers on your night stand.[210]

No matter what you may imagine, osteoporosis threatens 28 million Americans with more than half of postmenopausal women older than 50 walking around on thinning bones. This silent disease accounts for 1.5 million fractures annually and is a major cause for disability.[211-213] Your ethnic background also plays a role. If you are a Native American woman, your rate of bone loss is higher than in white women.[214] Asians are at greatest risk, while African American women make out the best of all.[215]

hear no evil, see no evil

It can even help you hear better. In a study of women's hearing, women on estrogen alone have significantly better hearing than women taking a combination of estrogen and progestins.[216] Although women of all ages have better hearing than men, they have a poorer capacity to hear at low frequencies as they enter menopause. More than 8 million women are estimated to have some degree of hearing trouble, and 2 million of those are able to hear, at best, only shouted words.[217] This loss of hearing may be due to changes in our brain's auditory reception, which is under the influence of ovarian hormones. Other research points to hypertension and dietary intake of saturated fat as a cause. [218,219]

Your eyes are another valuable asset that may be under the influence of estrogen. Glaucoma is a disease affecting drainage of fluid between the two chambers of the eye. As pressure within the eye builds up, sensitive nerve fibers that travel along the optic nerve become damaged, resulting in blindness. Women taking estrogen had lower intraocular pressures than women on eye drops alone, indicating a close relationship between the onset of menopause and the development of glaucoma.[220]

thanks for the sexy memories

As we age, our ability to remember and learn new things changes for the worse. Serotonin turnover drops and we are more prone to depression. In a study of postmenopausal women, estrogen was found to dramatically improve our ability to remember things we hear or read. Just a small dose can make the difference in how our brains retain information. Using magnetic resonance imaging, or MRI, scientists discovered estrogen can switch on neural circuits involved in memory, making them more flexible and malleable, despite our age.[314] This helps us to become more organized in our ability to process information and remember the telephone number for Aunt Betty's Poodle Parlor. It can boost short-term memory, improve reaction times and counter depression by rewiring our central nervous system.

When it comes to our sex life, estrogen is a woman's Viagra.™ Without it, our vagina begins to shrink and we develop urinary tract problems of incontinence, infection and irritation. Low or insufficient levels of estrogen can lead to bladder infections. Let me tell you about a former patient, Dena.

She was a tornado of a woman who bore and raised thirteen children. She never sat still. She talked as fast as she voided. By her own account, Dena sat on the toilet as little as possible. After urinating, she'd dash to her feet and be off to do something more important.

But then Dena developed what doctors call menopausal cystitis. Actually, she had symptoms of bladder problems all her life, but she could usually stave off infections by drinking tons of water and urinating often. Thanks to her strong abdominal muscles, she could write her name in the snow. But like most women who had children, Dena had a cystocele, or hernia of her bladder wall that held a small amount of urine. This gave her a weak vagina that allowed her bladder to fall down like a stack of dominos. Once this happened, her strong abdominal muscles were no longer effective in forcing the urine out. If you are interested in this topic, read the chapter on "How Menopause and Aging Affect Your Urologic Health" in my previous book "You Don't Have to Live With Cystitis." Suffice it to say estrogen not only strengthens our vagina, it can improve our mood and sex life so we can remember the position on page 54 of the Joy of Sex.[221-223]

the progesterone/progestin controversy

Progestins are synthetic drugs that share the ability to stimulate the progesterone receptor, yet that is where the similarity between the two ends. While progesterone helps support and maintain a pregnancy, progestins are used as a contraceptive, regulator of menstrual periods, protector of estrogen-stimulated endometrium and as anticancer therapy.[224] In fact, the effect of progestins in a woman's body are the opposite of the natural hormone progesterone. So why are progestins used in hormone replacement therapy?

This is a highly controversial area, and one which is undergoing extensive investigation and debate. But a few things are clear: progestins act similar to steroids in the body, altering our response to insulin.[39] Progestins can mimic, or potentiate the action of androgens, acting like a weaker version of testosterone on many tissues.[225] They can bind to cortisol receptors in white blood cells causing changes in your ability to fight infection.[226] None of this is a "good thing" if a woman is looking to restore the natural responses of progesterone in her body. Not only do progestins counteract the positive effects

Progestins increase the tension in the carotid artery that can lead to strokes

of estrogen on your heart, but they increase the tension in the carotid artery, which can lead to strokes.

From a weight gain standpoint, progestins and natural progesterone must plead guilty. By increasing insulin resistance in the body, they also inhibit the release of glucagon and growth hormone, favoring fat deposition and a bad lipid profile in a dose-dependent manner.[227] Progestins cause fluid retention, a less active bowel, breast tenderness, headaches and depression. So what choices are there if you want to protect your heart and your uterus?

It may surprise you to learn there are many options available today that make sense. A micronized version of progesterone, which has been available in Europe for the past 10 years, was approved for marketing in the US. Prometrium was evaluated in the Postmenopausal Estrogen/Progestin Intervention (PEPI) study and found to not only protect the lining of the uterus, but when used in combination with estrogen, raised the good cholesterol levels, which in turn protects the heart. In an earlier study, micronized estradiol and progesterone, when taken daily, quieted the endometrium within six months stopping all periods while improving a woman's lipid profile.[228] That's what I call protection and convenience!

baste don't marinate

The question of estrogen dosage is another area which has scientists scurrying to find an answer. Over the years, numerous types of estrogen have been developed and different ways to deliver them to the body. Although you may wear a perfect size 6, finding the right estrogen to fit your body is another matter as it is clear "one dose does NOT fit all." You can eat it, suck it, sniff it, rub it, inject it or stick it on. But despite all these routes, 10 to 25% of estrogen users have an insufficient bone response and 30 to 60% have a less than desirable clinical response when

it comes to their heart.[229] In a review by Dr. Bruno de
Lignieres, non-oral administration of estradiol, as in a
gel or patch, yielded the most promising results in
maintaining an optimal blood level of estradiol. By
checking estradiol levels, he determined that a concentration between 60 and 150pg/ml was sufficient to
offer all the benefits of estrogen therapy while
minimizing any side effects.[230] So there's no need to
marinate your body in high doses of estrogen when
just a little basting will do the trick.

hot flashes can make you fat

You're at a fancy restaurant and suddenly your
skin color matches the steamed lobster on your plate,
and you begin to sweat like one. Hot flashes, or that
trip to Tahiti you seem to take all by yourself, are the
most frequent complaint of women going through
menopause.[231] Although the exact physiologic reason
for its occurrence remains unknown, it appears to be
related to a change in our bodies' thermostat. As
estrogen levels fall, changes in the release of
leutenizing hormone cause a drop in the set point of
our thermoregulatory center. A hot flash is merely
the body's attempt to decrease our core body
temperature and restore temperature balance.[232] But a
hot flash has other effects on our body. We produce
almost 100% more norepinephrine under the
direction of the hypothalamus which constricts our
blood vessels, doubles the amount of free fatty acids
in the blood and increases the levels of LH.[233] Five
minutes later, ACTH is released by the pituitary in an
attempt to cool down the hypothalamus, and after
fifteen minutes cortisol increases in response to the
ACTH.[234] Remember, when cortisol levels go up, they
turn off your fat burning mechanisms and give the
green light to your intestines to open up the
floodgates for fat. Your omentum turns into a super
sponge slurping up the excess norepinephrine while
insulin directs free fatty acids to your hidden intra-

abdominal sites. Your waistline just moved up under your bustline. This is where estrogen comes in. Estrogen enhances the ability of our blood vessels to dilate by making nitric oxide available, which in effect, counteracts the vasoconstriction caused by too much norepinephrine.[235,236] It also counteracts the fat storing responses of insulin and cortisol. So keeping hot flashes under control can do more than keep your bed from turning into a swamp at night.

But not all hot flashes are due to lowering estrogen levels. As you can see in Table 8 there is a wide variety of conditions that can't respond to estrogen, so be sure to check with your doctor if estrogen therapy doesn't stop you from taking that unexpected trip to the Bahamas in your night shirt.

Table 8

non-menopausal causes for hot flashes

- Carcinoid syndrome
- Systemic mast cell disease
- Pheochromocytoma
- Medullary carcinoma of the thyroid
- Pancreatic islet cell tumors
- Renal cell carcinoma
- Neurologic flushing
- Emotional flushing
- Spinal cord injury
- Alcohol
- Drugs
- Food additives

show me the dark side

By now you might think we should dump estrogen into the drinking water of America! However, there is a dark side to taking hormones, and one you should know as an informed consumer.

the smoking gun

If you smoke, you shouldn't take estrogen. It's a simple fact. Smoking stimulates the formation of blood clots. Nearly 24 million women smoke cigarettes with an estimated 60,000 women dying annually from smoking-related heart disease.[237] The really good news is that women who stop smoking can reduce their risk of heart disease by 2.5% within a year. If you are a smoker, the most important lifestyle change you can make for yourself is to quit. And don't be afraid to ask for help or even to fail. Nicotine addiction is as potent a modulator of behavior as cocaine. By using a nicotine replacement program under a physician's guidance, you can double the odds of successfully quitting the habit. And if you need more encouragement, women who smoke have a far greater risk of ending up with that old, haggard wrinkled look on their face not even estrogen can help.[238] So if you can avoid smoking for three months, you are likely to become smoke free. And that means you can consider estrogen to help keep you healthy.

gallstones

Numerous studies have been done investigating the association between estrogen and gallstones. If you remember the woman at the beginning of this book, gallstones cause severe right upper abdominal pain which can radiate straight through to your back and up to your shoulder blade. There is evidence that estrogen promotes the formation of gallstones by increasing the ability of bile to precipitate or crystalize cholesterol. This in turn causes a sluggish gallbladder which doesn't empty efficiently. Remember, bile is necessary to break down fats in the foods we eat, especially saturated fats. It seems to make no difference whether the estrogen is taken orally or transdermally.[239,240] However, the risk of gallstones is very small among women on estrogen therapy.[241,242] It seems women stand a greater chance of undergoing surgery to remove their gallbladders because of symptoms mimicking gallbladder disease than for actual stone formation.[243,244]

endometrial cancer

Weekly alcohol consumption and decreased exercise increase your risk for endometrial cancer

The possibility that conjugated estrogens, the type derived from horse urine, could increase your risk of endometrial cancer resulted in two landmark studies in 1975. Ziel and Finkle reported that sodium estrone sulfate usage was associated with 50% of the cases found to have endometrial cancer.[245] In a much larger study, Smith and Prentice looked back at women with endometrial cancer and found a 4.5 times greater risk among estrogen only users.[246] This sparked a firestorm of controversy about estrogen which hasn't ceased to this day. But newer studies show a much more promising picture. Women who use estrogen and develop endometrial cancer have a much lower, less aggressive grade of tumor and a much higher cure rate than women who never use estrogen and develop cancer. The risk of death for a non-user was almost 7 times that of an estrogen user.[247] Several studies came to the same conclusion regardless of the dosage of estrogen.[248,249] Now a new study implicates weekly alcohol consumption and decreased exercise as the culprit. This increases the blood levels of estrogen and androstenedione, a male hormone that can be metabolized into estrone and then converted into estradiol.[250] The cure? If you take estrogen, you have to get off the couch and exercise and curtail any drinking. Even adding progestins for 10 days of the cycle only decreases but doesn't eliminate the risk for endometrial cancer. And there is a downside to this too–a relative, but small increased risk of breast cancer.[251]

breast cancer

Like endometrial cancer, women who take estrogen and develop breast cancer have smaller, less aggressive tumors than women without hormone therapy.[252] Researchers think that estrogen may have a direct inhibitory effect on established breast tumors, resulting in a more favorable outcome. If you consider the overall mortality risk for the average woman is much greater for cardiovascular disease (22%) than from breast cancer (3.3%), a woman will gain more useful years of life taking hormones even if she has a high risk of breast cancer.[253, 254] So why are women running scared?

lose the fear

Unfortunately, may doctors try to intimidate women by using the threat of cancer to get them to follow their proposed course of treatment. According to Dr. P.J. DiSaia, who studied breast cancer patients on hormones, estrogen therapy failed to "fuel the fire" of recurrent disease.[255] Instead, there is a "sea of emotion" when dealing with cancer. "Because freedom from recurrent breast cancer can never be guaranteed," he writes, " some women will develop recurrences regardless of hormone status. As a women you must realize that everything in medicine involves a risk/benefit analysis and only by being properly informed can you make decisions regarding estrogen."

Let's face it. We're all going to die, so it only makes sense to make the most of the time we have. Don't let your fear of death stop you from feeling the best you can. There's no guarantee that we have tomorrow. That's why today is a present.

natural therapies

Many women feel that taking estrogen solely to treat hot flashes is like using a cherry bomb to kill an ant! I couldn't agree more if this was the *only* benefit of estrogen. However, if after reading all the evidence in this chapter, you are still uncomfortable about estrogen, it would be unfair of me not to mention some very practical and worthwhile ways to manage the *symptoms* of menopause BEFORE your ovaries go two claws up!

> • Plant estrogens, known as isoflavone phytoestrogens, can be helpful in decreasing the number of hot flashes you experience when your estrogen levels are dropping. It takes about 80 gm of tofu or 50 mg of isolated isoflavones in capsule form to do this. In a study reported in the American Journal of Clinical Nutrition, these same vegetables were studied in combination with hormones. The great news is taking soy-derived phytoestrogens in combination with estradiol did not result in a dangerous buildup of the endometrium.[256] I eat one serving of soy a day and take 40 mg of isoflavones in capsule form daily with my estrogen. However, if you are hypothyroid, do not take any isoflavone supplements, as they may worsen your condition.

> • Physical exercise on a regular basis significantly lowers the number of hot flashes experienced, possibly due to effects on the neurotransmitters which regulate central thermoregulation.[257]

• Deep breathing can help to shorten the amount of time you spend flushing and may be of benefit in decreasing the frequency of hot flashes. Practice taking slow deep breaths involving your diaphragm whenever possible.

the secret of chicken soup

Grandmother really did know best when she gave you chicken soup to "feed a cold" but did you know it could control hot flashes? Arginine is an amino acid found in the gelatinous material extracted from bone marrow. It's what gives chicken soup its medicinal properties. The jelly stuff that congeals on your plate contains a growth factor which can slow down the rate of replication of viruses, but more importantly, arginine and vitamin E can block the atherosclerotic plaques that cause blood vessels to go into spasm and deprive your tissue of oxygen.[304] Arginine, especially L-arginine, restores the protective effects of cholecystokinin on the stomach lining.[305] It can also prevent damage to the kidneys by increasing the excretion of nitric oxide metabolites, which can cause scarring of the filtration units called glomeruli.[306]

Arginine helps wounds heal from surgery by stimulating the immune system in surgical patients.[307] But the most exciting thing I discovered was how well it worked to control and prevent hot flashes. The process that occurs in a hot flash results in blood vessels going into spasm due to signals coming from our central nervous system. Viagra™ works in much the same way. Nitric oxide can make blood vessels relax or dilate. However, we cannot produce nitric oxide in our bodies without arginine supplying the nitrogen. The discovery of arginine-derived nitric oxide was so important it resulted in the 1998 Nobel Prize in Medicine.

Nitric oxide levels depend upon a complex interaction between L-arginine and small estrogen doses. L-arginine stimulates growth hormone

Arginine lowers your blood pressure, handcuffs cholesterol and controls hot flashes

production and inhibits the effect of cortisol on our hormones.[308] Arginine lowers your blood pressure and can protect your heart by handcuffing cholesterol, that gunky stuff that turns arteries into grease-laden pipes. A diet rich in carbohydrates has very little arginine, while a protein rich diet has oodles of this amino acid. Soybeans, turkey and chicken contain large amounts of arginine. In fact, soy is exceptionally rich in arginine compared to animal sources. So try taking 500mg of L-arginine twice a day and forget about looking like a furnace.

what doesn't work

• Dong guai was found to be no more helpful than placebo or a protein diet in relieving menopausal symptoms after 24 months.[258]

• Vitamin E at doses of 800 IU daily had only a marginal effect on reducing the number of hot flashes when compared to a placebo.[259]

As you can see, I am "pro" estrogen in low doses for women when combined with a healthy diet and exercise. However, I do not support the use of continual progestin therapy in combination with estradiol, as studies have shown it to raise a woman's risk of breast cancer by 80% over 10 years.[316-318] Each of you must make a personal decision about hormone therapy. Think about the information in this chapter and discuss it with your doctor. In my newsletter, available online at **http://www.menopausediet.com**, I will keep you informed of the latest in research on this topic and others important to women. After all, you are the only one who can decide what is right for *you*.

chapter seven

why stress can make you fat

You're patiently waiting for a parking spot in a crowded shopping mall when a rogue automobile comes tearing down the aisle, swinging right into your slot. You hit the horn, start screaming and vow to flatten two tires on that sucker once you find ANOTHER spot! At that very moment you are getting fat!

Stress, especially chronic stress taxes your heart, scrambles your brain and sabotages your immune system from working like the national guard to protect your body against infection and cancer. But more importantly, even stressful thoughts can deprive your tissue of oxygen and the necessary chemicals to keep your hormones in balance.

to fight or flee : that is the question

Just imagine you're a gazelle frolicking on the Serengeti plains of Africa. Life is good and you don't have a care in the world. That is, until a lion shows up. Suddenly your heart takes the elevator to the top floor along with your blood pressure and you pass on being the blue plate special for the day and run like hell. During those few moments, your brain faxed your adrenals to squeeze out cortisol, norepinephrine and adrenaline or epinephrine to give you the energy for this life-or-death emergency. Once you are safe, your body "stands down," and resumes its normal function. Or at least that's how our bodies were designed.

Unfortunately, in our high stress society, we put ourselves through disaster training several times a day, which triggers these hormones to grab high-octane fat and quick burning glucose for energy to supply our brain, heart and muscles. And with that comes the necessity to store more fat. There's no question that cortisol increases fat deposition in one place, the worst place of all...the belly.

stress can break your heart

Menopausal women are the more fragile sex when it comes to their ability to handle stress, especially mental stress. While performing three mental stress tasks, womens' brains were studied by nuclear scanning while measurements were taken of their blood pressure. Postmenopausal women have significantly greater blood pressure reactivity than men or premenopausal women when under mental stress.[260] This is NOT a good thing. The presence of mental stress reduces the blood supply to the heart at lower heart rates than during exercise, giving a new meaning to the word "stress testing."[261] When researchers studied women who were stressed out in their day to day lives, or who felt tense, frustrated, sad and lonely, they were twice as likely to risk a heart attack in the following hour![262] If that wasn't enough, a ten year study of women who swallowed their anger but maintained a hostile attitude had higher plaque formation in their carotid arteries and could stroke out than women who expressed themselves and got on with life.[263] Despite the decrease in coronary heart disease (CHD) mortality in the US in the past 30 years, CHD kills nearly 500,000 American women each year, with African American women having a higher prevalence of CHD risk factors and a higher death rate at a younger age than white women.[264]

We put ourselves through disaster training several times a day

putting your ovaries in a twist

Stress packs a whollop throughout your whole body and can affect your ability to ovulate, a precious commodity during those waning years of menopause. By firing up your sympathetic nerve pathways, the celiac plexus, a major switching station behind the stomach, stocks up on norepinephrine and signals the ovaries to release the same neural transmitter. This accompanies an increase in testosterone and estradiol, causing precystic follicles to develop with a drop in ovulation.[265] Before you realize it, you've created a cyst, which can cause pain in your side and make you feel like weeping. When sheep are faced with a barking dog (audiovisual stress) or insulin-induced hypoglycemia (metabolic stress) they produce acute rises in adrenocortical hormone (ACTH), cortisol, epinephrine and norepinephrine which can only be turned off by high doses of estrogen.[266] As a menopausal women with lowering estrogen levels, you simply don't have enough estrogen reserve to combat your stress response hormonally. And if you spend sleepless nights worrying about things, you might as well be counting pounds instead of sheep.

sick and tired

We simply do not have enough estrogen reserve to combat stress

Long term stress not only causes weight gain but it does a number on your immune system. You become susceptible to colds and flus and feel just plain tired. Wounds take longer to heal because cortisol prevents the normal buildup of killer white cells in the body. Even just taking a test can stress you out and make you sick. Dental students were given wounds to the roof of their mouths three days before their final exam and again during summer vacation. (does this give you an idea of what professors think of their students?) Not surprisingly, the wounds took 40% longer to heal during the test time because of a

70% decline in the production of a particular type of white blood cell messenger RNA.[267] This same response was found in caretakers of Alzheimer patients, proving that psychological stress can make you a target for illness.[268]

who am I? where am I?

If you've ever spent hours looking for your keys, or that credit card bill that was due tomorrow, you may be experiencing some memory loss due to stress. Glucocorticoids, the adrenal steroid hormones secreted during stress, can damage the hippocampus or memory center of your brain by depriving the tissue of energy producing glucose.[269] It only takes 4 hours of stress to uncouple the neurons in your brain thanks to the plentiful receptors for corticosterone, the stress hormone in the hippocampus. This can affect your learning ability and may even cause brain cancer.[270] Repeated stress causes brain cells to shrink and can permanently damage nerve cells.[271] A recent study at McGill University in Quebec found that older people with high cortisol levels had smaller hippocampi and showed greater memory loss than their less-stressed peers. Women especially are more vulnerable to stress-induced memory loss than men. Stress hormones block the pituitary's ability to send signals to the ovary to ovulate and these same hormones make your ovaries less responsive. The net result is estrogen, leutenizing and follicle stimulating hormones are suppressed. Without estrogen, there is no control over damage from corticosterone in the brain.[272] No wonder you seem to be having a "senior moment" about those car keys.

fattening up your sleep cycle can trim your weight

You open your left eye and peek at the clock. It's 2 AM and you can't get back to sleep, so you turn on the TV just to hear the test pattern play white noise in the background. You feel unhappy and depressed - sort of out of sync with your life. Unfortunately, disturbances in your ability to sleep can cause you to gain weight.

Serotonin, that feel good hormone, is a precursor to melatonin, which is produced by the pineal gland in the brain, a pea size organ behind the hypothalamus. The role of melatonin is to help regulate your sleep, but women in menopause have low levels due to changes in their hormone status.[273] Sleep disturbances are common. Melatonin has other roles, and one of them is the regulation of glucose by the central nervous system in a non-insulin dependent manner.[274] When you sleep, melatonin levels go up in response to darkness and go down when your eyes are exposed to light. But if you are unable to stay asleep long enough, you disturb the glucose levels in your blood that keep your brain fed during the night.[275] Your body rhythm gets out of whack and this causes less growth hormone to be produced. Remember, growth hormone and estrogen mobilize fat in the body, while cortisol and insulin store fat. Growth hormone (GH) peaks during sleep just before you start to dream, so if you don't get several episodes of rapid eye movement sleep (REM) in a night, you can't produce sufficient GH and melatonin to keep blood glucose levels in check. In short, you get fat. Just in case you thought taking melatonin was the answer to burning the midnight oil - think again. Melatonin increases the production of somatostatin, a hormone that turns off glucagon and growth hormone production. It takes the rhythm of darkness and light in a 24 hour period to turn it back on.

Tossing and turning can make you fat

Several studies have looked at obesity and sleep disturbances and found that both depression and sleep alterations were signs of insulin resistance.[276-278] In particular, abdominal weight gain was confirmed by an increased waist-hip ratio due to high levels of cortisol directing fat storage to the abdomen instead of the thighs.[279] Tossing and turning all night consistently inhibits the ability of the body to produce GH-releasing hormone, which signals the body to produce GH and increases the amount of insulin-like growth factor-I. This is all corrected when sleep is restored.[280]

don't hold your breath

Another important medical problem, sleep apnea or breath holding, can happen when you don't get enough sleep. Studies have shown a strong link between a Buddha Belly and sleep apnea. It seems sleep is a very active metabolic time for us, and if we don't get enough oxygen during the night we can gain weight or prevent the loss of weight by reducing the production of growth hormone and estrogen. This changes your energy balance and insulin sensitivity creating a change in your brain's response to serotonin.[281] In a study of the relationship between lowered sympathetic nerve activity and obesity, researchers found that we become more sensitive to essential fatty acids when our serotonin levels drop and that makes you not only fat but depressed.[282,283]

stress busters

So, now that you realize how destructive stress can be in your life, what are you going to do about it? Here is what I found helpful:

> • **Laugh.** It may sound silly, but laughter not only supplies oxygen to your body, it creates movement. I am personally addicted to episodes of "Absolutely Fabulous" but I have been known to slip an occasional "Fawlty Towers" cassette into my player and roll on the floor in hysterics.

• **Sing.** The benefits of singing are numerous, especially if you learn to sing from your diaphragm (the part beneath your rib cage... not the one in your drawer!!) I especially recommend doing it in a foreign language so as to eliminate the embarrassment of not remembering the words.

• **Dance.** There is nothing more stress relieving than an attack of "Happy Feet." It doesn't matter what style you choose, just move and breathe and feel the rhythm of the music.

• **Walk.** Take 15 minutes a day to soak in the sunshine. Not only will you improve your mood but it can help you lose weight by adjusting your melatonin cycle and making you more responsive to insulin.[284]

• **Pose.** Just making yourself be still can help blow off steam. Yoga or meditation are ways to lower the stress hormones. For others, running helps them meditate in motion. If you're feeling stressed, assume the balance pose or T posture. Begin by standing comfortably, arms at your sides, and slowly fold forward from the hips. Extend your arms past your ears and bring your torso parallel to the ground. Simultaneously extend your left leg straight behind you. Breathe deeply and aim for stillness. Gently come back to your standing position and switch sides.

• **Primp.** Pamper yourself. Remember, you're worth every cent you earn or spend. Take a bubble bath, a steam shower or soak in a hot tub filled with flower petals.

• **Sleep.** Get to bed by 9:00 PM. Melatonin levels start to rise around 9:30 so pay attention to how much light you are exposed to in a 24 hour period. At least 9 hours of sleep are required by your body to reset your biological clock and improve your insulin sensitivity.

• **Inhale.** Pay attention to aromas. Cleopatra soaked the sails of her ship in fragrant oils to announce her approach to Rome. Try relaxing oils of ylang ylang, bergamot, tuberose, motia or orange soaked on a cotton ball. Inhaling a fragrance can stir pleasing memories which cause endorphins, the body's natural pain killers, to be released. Burn a candle or put a diffuser in your room. Just a few whiffs of lavender oil can lull you to sleep.

• **Pray.** Prayer-walking, also known as "walk-ing meditation" provides an easy way to be active and relieve stress. It can be a meandering saunter down a garden path or a brisk march around a track. The point is to walk with prayerful intentions realizing that your journey is an interior one.

Post inspirational quotes around your work area and be thankful for being alive. There's more to life than you'll ever realize and every day brings new chances to share.

chapter eight

nutritional support:
a helping hand

If you follow the concepts of The Menopause Diet, you should realize you are improving your vitamin balance by eating nutritionally dense foods. However, since you will be eliminating many of the "fortified" grains and starches, the addition of selected nutritional supplements is like buying collision insurance. So let's go over what nutrients may behave like an airbag in your diet.

- **Calcium** is essential for women in menopause to promote healthy bones and lower high blood pressure. It can reduce the risk of cancer of the colon, strokes and even kidney stones. In a study of dietary fat and calcium intakes, postmenopausal women ate more than the recommended amount of dietary fat while ignoring foods high in calcium.[285] Even the dietary intake of calcium in Chinese women was below the recommended daily allowance, putting them at risk for osteoporotic fractures.[286] Good sources are all dairy products except butter, lentils, most dark leafy greens and the soft bones of sardines. The easiest way to consume calcium is in mineral water. Supplementation with 800mg/d may prevent osteoporosis in postmenopausal women when given along with Vitamin D.[287] If you are concerned about bone loss, use a calcium supplement with bicarbonate as the anion or negative charged molecule.

You actually strengthen and increase the amount of bone production in your body by alkalinizing your system.[315] I take 750mg of calcium carbonate a day.

• **Folic acid**, one of the B vitamins, lowers blood levels of homocysteine, a risk factor for atherosclerotic disease. A simple deficiency of this vitamin can trigger 30 to 40% of the heart attacks and strokes suffered in America.[288] In a study of folate intake and its effect on homocysteine levels, researchers found the current RDA of 180 microg/d failed to maintain low levels of this amino acid and recommended an intake of 516 microg/d to decrease the levels of homocysteine in postmenopausal women.[289] Folic acid can also protect against cancer by altering DNA changes in your white blood cells. Good sources for folate are liver, nuts, lentils, spinach and other dark leafy greens, oranges and avocados. For the best availability of folate, choose fresh produce from a Farmer's market or the organic section of your grocery store.

• **Beta carotene**, a precursor of Vitamin A, is believed to reduce the risk of certain types of cancer. It's water soluble, which means if you take too much you'll wind up nourishing your toilet bowl. Food sources such as dark orange fruits and vegetables, like winter squash, pack an amazing amount of beta carotene into a single serving. As several foods containing beta carotene are high glycemic foods, I supplement my diet with 5000 iu a day.

• **Vitamin E** or d-alpha tocopherol is a powerful antioxidant which acts like a bug zapper to protect the first line of defense of any cell–

its membrane. Vitamin E, which is fat soluble, helps keep the good cholesterol high (HDL) while lowering the bad cho-lesterol (LDL) and can reduce the swelling from arthritis while slowing down the development of cataracts. Good sources are peanut butter, liver, leafy greens, soybeans and nuts. Dosages above 800iu may cause hypertension. As freezing of vegetables destroys the activity of vitamin E, it's best to eat fresh food sources. I use 200 iu daily in my diet.

• **Selenium** is a trace mineral that functions in concert with Vitamin E to scavenge free radicals and heavy metals. It is thought to help in the prevention of cancer. It's also important for thyroid function, as it aids in converting T4 to T3. Good sources include Brazil nuts, eggs, lean meats, seafood and legumes. Although the RDA for this mineral is 55mcg, I take 83mcg to insure adequate absorption.

• **Zinc** serves many functions in our body. The bitter metallic taste in your mouth when you eat iodinated table salt is caused by the interaction of zinc in your saliva with the iodine. This metal is important to carbohydrate, fat and protein metabolism and can assist your immune system in fighting a cold. Insulin-like growth factor (IGF-I) is a critical element in bone formation and protein metabolism. Low concentrations of zinc were found to cause low levels of IGF-I in healthy postmenopausal women.[290] In another study, animals switched from preferring carbohydrates to fat after developing a zinc deficiency.[291] Diets high in calcium or calcium containing supplements can reduce the absorption and balance in adults and have a direct effect on hip osteoporosis.[292,287] Foods high in zinc include meat and poultry (especially dark meat), shellfish and legumes. I routinely take 35 mg a day.

• **Vitamin C** has been viewed as the miracle vitamin, curing everything from the common cold to cancer in various doses. Ascorbic acid (Vitamin C) can reduce the risk of gallbladder disease and stones by altering the breakdown of cholesterol.[293-295] Vitamin C levels are associated with a reduction in heart disease and stroke.[296] Postmenopausal women who take at least 500mg of calcium a day with Vitamin C have better collagen formation in bone and tissue.[297] Good sources are fresh fruits, melons, strawberries, broccoli, sweet red and green peppers, tomatoes, brussels sprouts, cabbage and dark leafy greens like chard, kale, collards, spinach, mustard and turnips. The darker or brighter the green pigment, the greater the Vitamin C content. I take 350mg a day.

• **Magnesium** is a mineral which acts to balance the solubility of calcium in urine and tissues. It is vital to metabolism and activates more than 300 different enzymes in the body, particularly those that need the B vitamins for action. It helps to prevent tooth decay by binding calcium to teeth. Good sources are avocados, green vegetables, chocolate (70% cocoa), legumes, nuts and seeds. You should take half as much magnesium as calcium in your supplements, so I use 360mg a day to balance my calcium intake.

• **Vitamin D** is God's gift from sunshine. It regulates phosphorus and calcium metabolism which is important for strong bones.

Good sources are cod liver oil, dairy products, butter, eggs, liver, fish such as salmon and of course, sunshine. I only add 33 i.u of cholecalciferol (Vitamin D) to my diet.

• **Biotin** is a highly sulfur containing B vitamin which plays a key role in carbohydrate, fat and protein metabolism. It's what gives rotten eggs their odor! Biotin is important for healthy nails, hair and skin. Good sources are egg yolks, meats, liver, milk, nuts, legumes, peanut butter, chocolate and cauliflower. If you don't eat eggs, consider adding 33 mcg to your diet.

• **Pantothenic acid**, by its Greek name, means "do anything" and that's just about how it works. It's a key component to Coenzyme A which is important to your metabolism of carbohydrates, fats and proteins. Good sources are most fish but all food groups contain some pantothenic acid. I use 166 mg a day.

• **Riboflavin** is nature's way of giving you the benefits of niacin without the "hot flashes." It's an important B vitamin in the metabolism of tryptophan and has been found to help prevent migraines.[298] Riboflavin is water soluble and works with B6, folate and niacin to maintain the integrity of red blood cells. It also helps to metabolize carbohydrates, fats and proteins. Good sources are liver, eggs, milk, yogurt, cheese, dark green vegetables, spinach and broccoli. I take 66 mg a day.

• **Potassium** is an important mineral in maintaining fluid balance. It also helps our body breakdown carbohydrates and protein. Good sources include fruits, vegetables, dairy products, fish, lean meats and poultry. I take 50mg a day.

• **Chromium** helps to regulate cholesterol and fatty acid production by making the body more sensitive to insulin. It also aids in the digestion of protein. Good sources are un-peeled apples, oysters, nuts, peanut butter, liver and meat. I take 83 mcg in the form of an amino acid chelate.

• **Manganese** is a trace element that appears in a variety of plants and animals. Our bodies use it to activate enzymes that are important in the metabolism of glucose and fatty acids. Good sources are tea, leafy vegetables, nuts, fruits and legumes. I balance my diet with 41 mg.

• **Pyridoxine** or B6 is essential for the metabolism of protein as it helps to convert glycogen into glucose which can be used by your muscles for energy. It is an important cofactor in the regulation of 26 aminotrans-ferases, enzymes that regulate the proper path-ways for our neuroendocrine system. If you are deficient in B6, you may form kidney stones when you eat sugars such as fructose or galactose.[299] Women need higher doses of B6 than men because we lose more B6 in our urine.[313] Women taking birth control pills to control menopausal excess bleeding can become depleted of B6, which results in disturbances in the metabolism of tryptophan. This can cause depression, anxiety, decreased sex drive and impaired glucose tolerance.[300,301] B6 is important in lowering homocysteine levels in blood. Pyridoxal-5-phosphate, the liver metabolized form of B6, is the active component. However, if you have problems with gastric emptying, you may not be able to absorb B6 from standard vitamins unless it has been treated for absorption in the small intes-tine or duodenum. I take 20mg enteric coated tablets of Pyridoxal-5-Phosphate twice a day. If you are prone to herpetic outbreaks, don't take B6.

• **Iron deficiency** can alter cholesterol metabolism and predispose you to gallstone formation.[302] As menstruation becomes irregular, monthly blood loss can become severe, creating a deficiency. However, once menstruation stops, higher levels of iron become stored as serum ferritin, which has been shown to be a risk factor for coronary disease.[303] Sources of iron include liver, dried lentils, meat, poultry, broccoli, kale and spinach. Soy products can block the absorption of iron. You should discuss supplementation with your doctor as there are many variables to consider in finding the appropriate dosage for you.

• **Arginine** is an excellent way to manage hot flashes if you don't want to take estrogen. I take 500mg a day to balance my insulin response and to protect my heart, but you may need it twice a day. As this can increase the acidity in your body, it's best to take it with another amino acid, ornithine, so as not to stimulate any outbreaks of herpetic viruses.

As you can see, nutritional support is just another part of "The Menopause Diet" lifestyle. Since everyone can use a helping hand, I designed "Female Formula Stress Tabs" to insure you have all the vitamins and minerals necessary to keep your program on track. Look for information about ordering this supplement in the resource section of this book or online at

http://www.menopausediet.com

As always, make healthy food your mainstay, but for smart nutrition insurance the right supplements make sense too.

chapter nine

menopause:
how to chart your own
personal journey

Trust me. This next step isn't going to hurt one
little bit. All you need is a tape measure to start
yourself off on your own personal journey to a
slimmer, more vivacious body. So close the door—
you don't need any Peeping Toms here and let's get
started.

calculating body mass index

Remember that weight is not the factor which
determines how healthy you are, but rather three
measurements: Body Mass Index, waist circumference and percent body fat. Its easy to measure your
waistline—just place the tape around the smallest part
of your abdomen above your belly button and below
your lowest rib. Go to the chart on the next page and
write down your waistline in inches. Now the next
two figures are a bit more complicated. To determine
your body mass index, you need to take your height
and convert it into inches and then meters squared.
The chart makes it easier. Now go weigh yourself.
Don't worry. I won't look.

I've included detailed instructions in the chart to
help you complete your profile. To determine your
percent body fat, I highly recommend the new electronic scale by Tanita or the hand held device by
Omron. When I used charts, I underestimated my
actual body fat by several pounds. Both devices emit
a low electrical current that calculates both the percent and actual pounds of fat on your body. Skin

calipers can also give you an accurate reading. The gold standard involves submersion in water to determine your precise amount of body fat. Since I am "water soluble" I prefer the electronic scale read-ings to keep track of my progress.

Now, if you want to know your basal metabolic rate or BMR (how many calories you burn just sitting) multiply your weight in pounds by 11. Add between 400 and 600 calories for mild to intense exercise and routine physical activity and you have a rough idea of how many 250 calorie meals you need in a day just to maintain your weight. Once you are armed with this information, you are ready to proceed to the next step.

body mass index

	21	22	23	24	25	26	27	28	29	30
5'0"	107	112	118	123	128	133	138	143	148	158
5'1"	111	116	122	127	132	137	143	148	153	158
5'2"	115	120	126	131	136	142	147	153	158	164
5'3"	118	124	130	135	141	146	152	158	163	169
5'4"	122	128	134	140	145	151	157	163	169	174
5'5"	126	132	138	144	150	156	162	168	174	180
5'6"	130	136	142	148	155	161	167	173	179	186
5'7"	134	140	146	153	159	166	172	178	185	191
5'8"	138	144	151	158	164	171	177	184	190	197
5'9"	142	149	155	162	169	176	182	189	196	203
5'10"	146	153	160	167	174	181	188	195	202	207
5'11"	150	157	165	172	179	186	193	200	208	215

1. Waist   _____inches
                                 Goal: Under 30 inches

2. Height   _____inches
                                 (multiply feet by 12 and add
                                 the rest as inches)

_____ meters^2 To convert to meters, multiply
                                 inches by 0.0254 then multiply
                                 that number against itself

                                 *Example 62 inches x 0.0254=1.5748
                                 x 1.5748=2.479 meters^2*

3. Weight   _____pounds To convert to
                                 kilograms, divide by 2.2
                                 _____kg

4. BMI = kg/m^2 _____ Simply take #3 divided
                                 by #2
                                 Goal: Under 25 kg/m^2

5. Percent body fat _____
                                 Goal: Under 25%

6. BMR =   _____ calories (weight in
                                 pounds x 11)

Add 400/600/1000 calories for degree of exercise,
routine physical activity and divide by 250 for the
number of mini meals in a day to maintain your
weight.

Calories/250 =   _____ mini meals/day

the family tree

I always asked my patients about the risks hiding in their family tree, specifically what illnesses occurred and the cause of any family member's death. More than 3,000 ailments are known to be inherited, including heart disease, cancer, diabetes, arthritis, Alzheimer's, even alcoholism, depression, thyroid disease and schizophrenia. Take time to fill this form out for both sides of your family and make copies for your children. It will make your motivation even stronger for losing weight and staying healthy.

old mother hubbard

I always clean out my cupboards on days when my hormones are really low, usually just before my period. It seems changes in serotonin cause an obsessive cleaning nature in women at this time, so take advantage of the situation and remove temp-tation, in the form of high glycemic carbohydrates from your shelves.

> • Designate a specific cupboard just for your own food items and place any cereals or bread in another cupboard for your family to use.

> • Replace cooking oils with olive oil, canola and peanut oil.

> • Stock up on spices and teas and get rid of cans of vegetables you've been saving since the beginning of the world.

> • Check labels for corn syrup or MSG and eliminate them from your personal cup-board.

Once you've got this situation in hand, let's deal with the shopping list.

your family health history

This blank genogram has room for only your own family history. But you can photo copy the page, add your spouse's family, and combine the two for your children's full health history. Squeeze in extra names, of course, if you have an especially large family. When your genogram is complete, give your doctor a copy for your medical files and make separate copies for your spouse's and children's files. Store another copy for each of your children and update it periodically.

Name of person submitting genogram _____

Date _____

Address _____

grand-
parents   ■ name: ● n: ■ n: ● n:

aunts,   n: n: n: n: n: n:
uncles,
parents

                    ■   ●

siblings your name: n: n:

after entering your relatives names, list birthdate, death date, ailments and cause of death
- *female*   ⌐⌐ *married*
- *male*

to market to market

Copy the list of high glycemic carbohydrates on page 46 and keep them with you in the grocery store. It's important in starting The Menopause Diet that you understand which carbohydrates have the ability to raise your blood sugar higher than the Empire State Building if you want to lose weight.

• Choose a wide variety of produce and try to avoid frozen or canned vegetables.

• Compare the grams of carbohydrates that come from sugar in any reduced fat dairy products versus the full fat versions to be certain you're not substituting sugar for fat.

• Lean meats usually come from the loin, so choose filet, pork loin and sirloin instead of ribs and heavily marbled meats.

• Select fish that is fresh, not frozen whenever possible and try to include at least one serving of tuna or salmon each week in your meal plan.

• If you're looking for additional non-fat protein sources, purchase whey and soy protein powders to add to soups, mayonnaise and dressings.

• Corn syrup is contained in an amazing number of soups and drinks, including orange juice concentrate, so be certain to read the labels before putting any new products into your cart.

• Purchase low fructose energy bars and keep one in your purse at all times so you don't accidentally skip a meal. It's saved me from many a munchy madness attack that would have overdrawn my carbohydrate reserve account.

eating out

Portion control is probably the hardest part of eating out, with today's restaurants vying to win the Gordita Grande award when it comes to a main course. The simplest way to overcome this is to order two appetizers and request steamed vegetables as a side dish. Don't forget to eat a salad but demurely pass on the bread. The only time I have dessert is in a restaurant and I treat myself to the most appetizing one on the menu. Remember, the composition of the previous meal affects your next one, so don't be afraid to make an occasional withdrawal on that carbohydrate account.

urge to splurge

You've been great on The Menopause Diet but you're dying for some rice or bread. Can you eat it? Of course. You can do anything you want. But here is how I dealt with the occasional craving. I prepared as much of the food as my eyes told me I wanted, then put the entire serving on my plate along with my protein, fat and low glycemic carbs. I only allowed myself one high glycemic food at a meal every three days. It seemed after a few mouthfuls I didn't need any more to satisfy my urge to splurge. So don't deny yourself any food on the shopping list if you have a craving for it. **Just remember - each time you eat a high glycemic carb it's like putting 3 tablespoons of corn syrup in your mouth.**

charting your progress

Don't become obsessed about daily weight checks. Fluid levels fluctuate daily in your body and you can lose or gain a pound without having metabolized any fat. I recommend you weigh yourself once a week at the same time of day and take an inventory of your waistline every week. Notice how your clothes fit instead of where the needle on the scale is bouncing. It's a much better indicator of losing fat. Write down your weekly values and compare them after one month. I think you'll be pleased with the results you've achieved by not starving or denying yourself.

a final word

The Menopause Diet Plan will help you regain the vitality and shape of your youth without the need for pills or surgery. But more importantly, it can prolong your life by preventing the damage to your body from uncontrolled blood sugar that can lead to heart disease, strokes and cancer. So take the time to applaud yourself for living better than ever before and let the new balance in your life lead to a more healthy, beautiful and loving you.

appendix a
resources for living

the menopause diet website

If you are interested in learning more about the impact of diet on menopause, visit my website at

www.menopausediet.com

where you will find up to date news articles, discussions about the latest scientific research, a newsletter just for menopausal women and products of interest to us. You can order personally autographed copies of "The Menopause Diet," "The Menopause Diet Mini Meal Cookbook," "The Menopause Diet Daily Journal," motivational audio tapes along with my nutritional supplements "Female Formula Stress Tabs" and "Pyridoxal-5 Phosphate" by calling

1-800-554-3335 in the United States

or

310 471-2375
if you do not have access to the internet.

Share your personal experience with The Menopause Diet Plan on my message board and swap recipes and support with each other. It can be just the helping hand you need!

female formula stress tabs
60 tablets

Two tablets contain:

Beta Carotene	5000 i.u.
D-alpha Tocopherol Acetate	200 i.u.
Sodium Selenite	83 mcg
Zinc Gluconate	35 mg
Vit. C (from ascorbyl palmitate and ascorbic acid)	350 mg
Calcium Carbonate	750 mg
Magnesium Hydroxide	360 mg
Vit. D3 (cholecalciferol)	33 i.u.
Biotin	33 mcg
D-Calcium Pantothenate	166 mg
Riboflavin	66 mg
Potassium Chloride	50 mg
Chromium (amino acid chelate)	83 mcg
Manganese Gluconate	41 mg

pyridoxal-5-phosphate
30 tablets

One tablet contains:

Pyridoxal-5-Phosphate (enteric coated)	20mg

All supplements are 100% natural and free of yeast, corn, sugar, starch, soy, flavors, colors, preservatives, wheat or milk derivatives. All orders are shipped Priority Mail.

body fat monitors

The Tanita Body Fat Monitor/Scale is available at Macy's and other large department stores. The scale measures both weight and body fat in 30 seconds and is programmable for up to four people. It retails for $149.95.

Omron makes a portable hand held body fat analyzer that works on the same principle as the Tanita model. It retails for $129.95 at The Sharper Image and several other electronic stores.

- Call 1-800-634-4350 for a distributor near you.

spices

Purchasing new, exotic spices can lend a real zip to foods while keeping the fat low. One of the best sources is Penzeys Spice catalog. You can order their catalog on line at:
- Penzeys Spices
www.penzeys.com
414 679-7207.

For Allepo, pasilla and ancho chili powder, Dean and Deluca is an excellent resource. You can order online at:
- Dean and Deluca
www.dean-deluca-napavalley.com
707 967-9880.

Other sources for exotic spices are:
- Kalustyan
123 Lexington Ave
New York, NY 10016
212 685-3451

- Sultan's Delight
P.O. Box 090302
Brooklyn, NY 11209
800 852-6844   718 745-6844   Fax 718 745-2563

• The Spice House
1031 N. Old World Third St
Milwaukee, WI 53203
414 272-0977

teas

One of my favorite teas is made by Bernardaud's
of France. It's a caramel tea and is rich in flavor, even
when laced with a little milk. You can order it from:

• La Cucina Rustica
cyberbaskets.com/cbdocs/items/be9003c.htm
9950 West Lawrence Avenue, Suite 202
Schiller Park, IL 60176 USA
800 796-0116 – Customer Service Department

Stash makes a Mango Passion Fruit tea available
in grocery stores and Ceylon Passion has a delightful
Passion Fruit Papaya tea combination. A mixture of
black teas with fruit extract, they make delightful iced
teas. All are caffeine free and available in your grocery
store.

Tejava is a delicious micro brewed tea made entire-
ly from the top leaves of each branch picked only from
May through October. If you can't find it in your
grocery store, call 1-800-4-GEYSER

tomatoes

There is nothing better than fresh tomatoes, but
the organic canned tomatoes seasoned with sea salt
by Muir Glen do well in a pinch. If you don't find
them in your grocery store, call or write

• Muir Glen
P.O. Box 1498
Sacramento, California
707 778-7801
www.muirglen.com has a store locator on the site

recumbent bikes

To find a distributor for the BikeE CT 2.0, call:

- BikeE
1-800-231-3136
5125 S W Hout
Corvallis, Oregon 97333
It retails for $650.

pilates®

If you're looking for books, videos and equipment in order to perform Pilates® contact:

- Current Concepts
1-800-240-3539

They have several books available. Be sure and ask for this one:

- *Body Control Pilates* by Lynne Robinson and Gordon Thomson, BainBridge Books, 1998

Here are other resources for this exercise program:

- PhysicalMind Institute
1-800-505-1990

- Pilates Studio
1-800-474-5283
www.pilates-studio.com
They sell a foldable home exercise reformer for stretching

To get started on exercising, just go to any bookstore and stand in front of the health and fitness section. You will be amazed at how many ways you can tone and firm your body.

I recommend the following books for their clean, simple approach to understanding weight training and body shaping.

- *Body Shaping*
by Michael Yessis, PhD.,
Rodale Press, 1994

- *Callanetics*
by Callan Pinckney,
Perigee Books, 1997

- *Power Yoga*
by Beryl Bender Birch,
Fireside, 1995

- *A Woman's Book of Strength*
by Karen Andes,
Perigee Books, 1995

If you are interested in reading about the health benefits of arginine, pick up this book:

- *The Arginine Solution*
by Robert Fried Ph.D.
and Woodson Merrell, MD.,
Warner Books, 1999

There is only one book every person who has ever suffered from kidney stones should have in their home health library:

- *The Kidney Stones Handbook*,
Gail Savitz and Stephen Leslie, M.D.,
1999 Four Geez Press
1-800-2kidney
916 781-3440
1911 Douglass Blvd #85
Roseville, Ca 95661
ggolomb@ns.net

If you want to try Prayer-walking, read this book:

• *The Complete Guide to Prayer-Walking*
by Linus Mundy, Crossroads Publications, 1997

These books on breathing will give you a practical guide to deep relaxation and much more:

• *The Breathing Book*
by Donna Farhi,
Owl Books, 1996

• *The Tao of Natural Breathing*
by Dennis Lewis,
Mountain Wind Publishing, 1997

• *Conscious Breathing*
by Gay Hendricks, Ph.D.,
Bantam Books, 1995

This book by Mary Shomon, About.com Thyroid Guide, will open your eyes to the effect thyroid problems can have on weight gain, depression and fatigue. Told from her own personal experience as a patient.

• *Living Well With Hypothyroidism*
by Mary Shomon
HarperCollins/Avon/WholeCare, 2000
http://www.thyroid-info.com/booktoc.htm

Finally, a catalogue just for us "Menopausal Mommas." Full of devices, clothing, lotions and everything you could possibly need:

• As We Change
1-800-203-5585
aswechange.com

appendix b
references

1. Kuczmarski, R., *et al.*, *Increasing prevalence of overweight among US adults: the National Health and Nutrition Examination Surveys, 1960-1991.* JAMA, 1994. **272**: p. 205-211.

2. LaCroix, A. *and e. al*, *Healthy Aging: A Woman's Issue.* West. J. Med., 1997. **167**(Oct): p. 220-232.

3. Ulrich, L., *Lipids and women's health, ed.* G. Redmond. 1991, New York: Springer-Verlag. 66-79.

4. de Aloysio, D., *et al.*, *Premenopause-dependent changes.* Gynecol Obstet Invest, 1996. **42**(2): p. 120-7.

5. Geary, N., *Estradiol and the control of eating.* Appetite, 1997. **29**(3): p. 386.

6. Ganesan, R., *The aversive and hypophagic effects of estradiol.* Physiol Behav, 1994. 55(2): p. 279-85.

7. Petroianu, A., *Gallbladder emptying in perimenopausal women.* Med Hypotheses, 1989. **30**(2): p. 129-30.

8. Lam, W.F., *et al.*, *Influence of hyperglycemia on the satiating effect of CCK in humans.* Physiol Behav, 1998. **65**(3): p. 505-11.

9. Ortega, R.M., *et al.*, *Differences in diet and food habits between patients with gallstones and controls.* J Am Coll Nutr, 1997. **16**(1): p. 88-95.

10. Attili, A.F., *et al.*, *Diet and gallstones in Italy: the cross-sectional MICOL results.* Hepatology, 1998. **27**(6):p.1492-8.

11. Caroli-Bosc, F.X., *et al.*, *Cholelithiasis and dietary risk factors: an epidemiologic investigation in Vidauban, Southeast France. General Practitioner's Group of Vidauban.* Dig Dis Sci, 1998. **43**(9): p. 2131-7.

12. Gazizova, R.R., A.V. Novikova, and M.A. Vinogradova, *Age-related features of inflammatory and immune responses of the gastric mucosa in women with chronic gastritis.* Patol Fiziol Eksp Ter, **1995**(4): p. 32-4.

13. Konturek, J.W., *et al.*, *Physiological role of cholecystokinin in gastroprotection in humans.* Am J Gastroenterol, 1998. **93**(12): p. 2385-90.

14. Nilsson, P., *et al.*, *Social and biological predictors of early menopause: a model for premature aging.* J Intern Med, 1997. **242**(4): p. 299-305.

15. Wilson, J. and D. Foster, *Williams Textbook of Endocrinology.* 8 ed. 1992, Philadelphia: W.B. Saunders.

16. Rosano, G., *et al.*, *Syndrome X in women is associated with estrogen deficiency.* Eur Heart J, 1995. **16**(5): p. 610-14.

17. Spencer, C.P., I.F. Godsland, and J.C. Stevenson, *Is there a menopausal metabolic syndrome?* Gynecol Endocrinol, 1997. **11**(5): p. 341-55.

18. Colombel, A. and B. Charbonnel, *Weight gain and cardiovascular risk factors in the post-menopausal women.* Hum Reprod, 1997. **12** Suppl 1: p. 134-45.

19. Gensini, G.F., M. Comeglio, and A. Colella, *Classical risk factors and emerging elements in the risk*

profile for coronary artery disease. Eur Heart J, 1998. **19** Suppl A: p. A53-61.

20. Goodman, M.T., *et al., The association of diet, obesity, and breast cancer in Hawaii.* Cancer Epidemiol Biomarkers Prev, 1992. **1**(4): p. 269-75.

21. Legato, M.J., *Cardiovascular disease in women: gender-specific aspects of hypertension and the consequences of treatment.* J Womens Health, 1998. **7**(2): p. 199-209.

22. Maurer, K.R., *et al., Risk factors for gallstone disease in the Hispanic populations of the United States.* Am J Epidemiol, 1990. **131**(5): p. 836-44.

23. Large, V. and P. Arner, *Regulation of lypolysis in humans. Pathophysiological modulation in obesity, diabetes and hyperlipidaemia.* Diabetes Metab, 1998. **24**(5): p. 409-18.

24. Anate, M., A. Olatinwo, and A. Omesina, *Obesity– an overview.* West Afr J Med, 1998. **17**(4): p. 248-54.

25. Gannon, L. and J. Stevens, *Portraits of menopause in the mass media.* Women Health, 1998. **27**(3): p. 1-15.

26. Carey, D.G., *et al., Abdominal fat and insulin resistance in normal and overweight women: Direct measurements reveal a strong relationship in subjects at both low and high risk of NIDDM.* Diabetes, 1996. **45**(5): p. 633-8.

27. Goldsmith, H., *The Omentum.* 1990, New York: Springer-Verlag.

28. Bjorntorp, P., *The regulation of adipose tissue distribution in humans.* Int J Obes Relat Metab Disord, 1996. **20**(4): p. 291-302.

29. Bronnegard, M., P. Arner, and L. Hellstrom, *et al., Glucocorticoid receptor messenger ribonucleic acid in*

different regiosn of human adipose tissue. Endocrinol, 1990. **127**: p. 1689-1696.

30. Iannoli, P., *et al., Glucocorticoids upregulate intestinal nutrient transport in a time-dependent and substrate-specific fashion.* Gastrointest Surg, 1998. **2**(5): p. 449-57.

31. Bongain, A., V. Isnard, and J.Y. Gillet, *Obesity in obstetrics and gynaecology.* Eur J Obstet Gynecol Reprod Biol, 1998. **77**(2): p. 217-28.

32. Samojlik, E., M. Kirschner, and D. Silber, *et al., Elevated production and metabolic clearance rates of androgens in morbidly obese women.* J Clin Endocrinol Metab, 1984. **59**: p. 949.

33. Kirschner, M. and J. Jacobs, *Combined ovarian and adrenal vein catheterization to determine the site of androgen overproduction in hirsute women.* J Clin Endocrino Metab, 1971. **1**(33): p. 199.

34. Barbieri, R., *Adipose Tissue and Reproduction.* Prog Reprod Biol Med, ed. R. Frisch. Vol. 14. 1990, Basel: Karger. 42-57.

35. Lemieux, S., *et al., A single threshold value of waist girth identifies normal-weight and overweight subjects with excess visceral adipose tissue.* Am J CLin Nutr, 1996. **64**: p. 685-93.

36. Lyu, L.C., *et al., Relationship of body fat distribution with cardiovascular risk factors in healthy Chinese.* Ann Epidemiol, 1994. **4**(6): p. 434-44.

37. Panotopoulos, G., *et al., Weight gain at the time of menopause.* Hum Reprod, 1997. **12** Suppl 1: p. 126-33.

38. Stevenson, J.C., *et al., HRT mechanisms of action: carbohydrates.* Int J Fertil Menopausal Stud, 1994. **39**(Suppl 1): p. 50-5.

39. Gaspard, U.J., J.M. Gottal, and F.A. van den Brule, *Postmenopausal changes of lipid and glucose metabolism: a review of their main aspects.* Maturitas, 1995. **21**(3):p. 71-8.

40. Wild, R., P. Painter, and P. Coulson, *et al., Lipoprotein lipid concentrations and cardiovascular risk in women with polycystic ovarian syndrome.* J Clin Endocrinol Metab, 1985. **61**: p. 946.

41. Rexrode, K., *et al., Abdominal adiposity and coronary heart diease in women.* JAMA, 1998. **280**: p. 1843-1848.

42. Williams, M.J., *et al., Regional fat distribution in women and risk of cardiovascular disease.* Am J Clin Nutr, 1997. **65**(3): p. 855-60.

43. Harris, M., *Epidemiological correlates of NIDDM in Hispanics, whites and blacks in the US population.* Diabetes Care, 1991. **14**(Suppl 3): p. S639-S648.

44. Gavin, J., *The role of the gastrointestinal tract and alpha-glucosidase inhibition in Type II diabetes.* Drug Benefits Trends, 1996(Supp 8E): p. 18-26.

45. Jarrett, R., H. Keen, and J. Fulley, *et al., Worsening to diabetes in men with impaired glucose tolerance (borderline diabetes).* Diabetologia, 1979. **16**: p. 25-30.

46. Redberg, R.F., *Coronary artery disease in women: understanding the diagnostic and management pitfalls.* Medscape Womens Health, 1998. **3**(5): p. 1.

47. Wenger, N.K., *The High Risk of CHD for Women: Understanding Why Prevention Is Crucial.* Medscape Womens Health, 1996. **1**(11): p. 6.

48. Kahn, H.S., L.M. Tatham, and C.W. Heath, Jr., *Contrasting factors associated with abdominal and peripheral weight gain among adult women.* Int J Obes Relat Metab Disord, 1997. **21**(10): p. 903-11.

49. Bresnick, J. and T. Hanlon, *Custom tailored hormone therapy,* in Prevention. 1995. p. 65-73.

50. Knight., L., *et al., Delayed gastric emptying and decreased antral contractility in normal premenopausal women compared with men.* Am J Gastroenterol, 1997. **92**(6): p. 968-75.

51. Weber, E. and H.J. Ehrlein, *Relationships between gastric emptying and intestinal absorption of nutrients and energy in mini pigs.* Dig Dis Sci, 1998. **43**(6): p. 1141-53.

52. Raskin, P., *et al., Abnormal alpha cell function in human diabetes: the response to oral protein.* Am J Med, 1978. **64**(6): p. 988-97.

53. Wagner, R. and J. Warkany, *Untersuchungen uber den zuckerbildenden Wert der Gemuse in der Diabetikerkost.* Z Kinderheilk, 1927. **44**: p. 322.

54. Crapo, P., G. Reaven, and J. Olefsky, *Plasma glucose and insulin responses to orally administered simple and complex carbohydrates.* Diabetes, 1976. **25**: p. 741-747.

55. Wolever, T.M., *et al., Glycemic index of foods in individual subjects.* Diabetes Care, 1990. **13**(2): p. 126-32.

56. Jenkins, D., T. Wolever, and R. Taylor, *Glycemic index of foods: a physiological basis for carbohydrate exchange.* Am J Clin Nutr, 1981. **34**: p. 362-6.

57. Juliano, B.O., *et al., Properties of Thai cooked rice and noodles differing in glycemic index in noninsulin-dependent diabetics [published erratum appears in Plant Foods Hum Nutr 1990 Jul;40(3):231-2].* Plant Foods Hum Nutr, 1989. **39**(4): p. 369-74.

58. Wolever, T., *et al., Glycaemic index of 102 complex carbohydrate foods in patients with diabetes.* Nutr Res, 1994. **14**: p. 651-669.

59. Gannon, M. and F. Nuttall, *Factors affecting interpretation of postprandial glucose and insulin areas.* Diabetes Care, 1987. **10**: p. 759-763.

60. Melanson, K., *et al., Blood glucose and hormonal response to small and large meals in healthy young and old women.* J Gerontol: Biol Sc, 1998. **53A**: p. 4.

61. Wolever, T.M., *The glycemic index.* World Rev Nutr Diet, 1990. **62**: p. 120-85.

62. Nuttall, F., *et al., Effect of protein ingestion on the glucose and insulin response to a standardized oral glucose load.* Diabetes Care, 1984. **7**: p. 465-470.

63. Smith, G.P. and J. Gibbs, *Are gut peptides a new class of anorectic agents?* Am J Clin Nutr, 1992. **55**(1 Suppl): p. 283S-285S.

64. Welch, I., *et al., Duodenal and ileal lipid suppresses postprandial blood glucose an dinsulin responses in man: possible implications for the dietary managment of diabetes mellitus.* Clin Sci, 1987. **72**: p. 209-216.

65. Collier, G., T. Wolever, and D. Jenkins, *Concurrent ingestion of fat and reduction in starch content impairs carbohydrate tolerance to subsequent meals.* Am J Clin Nutr, 1987. **45**: p. 963-969.

66. Wolever, T.M. and C. Bolognesi, *Prediction of glucose and insulin responses of normal subjects after consuming mixed meals varying in energy, protein, fat, carbohydrate and glycemic index.* J Nutr, 1996. **126**(11): p. 2807-12.

67. Jenkins, D., *et al., Metabolic effects of a low-glycemic-index diet.* Am J Clin Nutr, 1987. **46**(6): p. 968-75.

68. Jenkins, D., T. Wolever, and G. Buckley, *et al., Low glycemic index starchy foods in the diabetic diet.* AM J

Clin Nutr, 1988. **48**: p. 248-254.

69. Jenkins, D., *et al.*, *Nibbling versus gorging: metabolic advantages of increased meal frequency.* N Engl J Med, 1989. **321**(14): p. 929-34.

70. Jenkins, D.J., *et al.*, *Low glycemic index: lente carbohydrates and physiological effects of altered food frequency.* Am J Clin Nutr, 1994. **59**(3 Suppl): p. 706S-709S.

71. Leibowitz, S.F., A. Akabayashi, and J. Wang, *Obesity on a high-fat diet: role of hypothalamic galanin in neurons of the anterior paraventricular nucleus projecting to the median eminence.* J Neurosci, 1998. **18**(7): p. 2709-19.

72. Jenkins, D., *et al.*, *"Nibbling versus gorging": metabolic advantages of increased meal frequency.* N Eng J Med, 1989. **321**: p. 929-34.

73. Himaya, A. and J. Louis-Sylvestre, *The effect of soup on satiation.* Appetite, 1998. **30**(2): p. 199-210.

74. Wolever, T.M., *et al.*, *Second-meal effect: low-glycemic-index foods eaten at dinner improve subsequent breakfast glycemic response.* Am J Clin Nutr, 1988. **48**(4): p. 1041-7.

75. Parodi, P.W., *The French paradox unmasked: the role of folate.* Med Hypotheses, 1997. **49**(4): p. 313-8.

76. Drewnowski, A., *et al.*, *Diet quality and dietary diversity in France: implications for the French paradox.* J Am Diet Assoc, 1996. **96**(7): p. 663-9.

77. Hercberg, S., *et al.*, *Vitamin status of a healthy French population: dietary intakes and biochemical markers.* Int J Vitam Nutr Res, 1994. **64**(3): p. 220-32.

78. Monneuse, M.O., F. Bellisle, and G. Koppert,

Eating habits, food and health related attitudes and beliefs reported by French students. Eur J Clin Nutr, 1997. **51**(1): p. 46-53.

79. Chatenoud, L., *et al.*, *Whole grain food intake and cancer risk.* Int J Cancer, 1998. **77**(1): p. 24-8.

80. La Vecchia, C. and A. Tavani, *Fruit and vegetables, and human cancer.* Eur J Cancer Prev, 1998. **7**(1): p. 3-8.

81. Michaud, C., *et al.*, *Food habits, consumption, and knowledge of a low-income French population.* Sante Publique, 1998. **10**(3): p. 333-47.

82. Jeffery, R.W. and S.A. French, *Epidemic obesity in the United States: are fast foods and television viewing contributing?* Am J Public Health, 1998. **88**(2): p. 277-80.

83. Larson, D.E., *et al.*, *Dietary fat in relation to body fat and intraabdominal adipose tissue: a cross-sectional analysis.* Am J Clin Nutr, 1996. **64**(5): p. 677-84.

84. Ginsberg, H.N., *et al.*, *Effects of reducing dietary saturated fatty acids on plasma lipids and lipoproteins in healthy subjects: the DELTA Study, protocol 1.* Arterioscler Thromb Vasc Biol, 1998. **18**(3): p. 441-9.

85. O'Bryne, D.J., S.F. O'Keefe, and R.B. Shireman, *Low-fat, monounsaturate-rich diets reduce susceptibility of low density lipoproteins to peroxidation ex vivo.* Lipids, 1998. **33**(2): p. 149-57.

86. Low, C., E. Grossman, and B. Gumbiner, *Potentiation of effects of weight loss by monunsaturated fatty acids in obese NIDDM patients.* Diabetes, 1996. **45**: p. 569-575.

87. O'Byrne, D.J., D.A. Knauft, and R.B. Shireman, *Low fat-monounsaturated rich diets containing high-oleic peanuts improve serum lipoprotein profiles.* Lipids, 1997. **32**(7): p. 687-95.

88. Trautwein, E.A., *et al.*, *Effect of dietary fats rich in lauric, myristic, palmitic, oleic or linoleic acid on plasma, hepatic and biliary lipids in cholesterol-fed hamsters.* Br J Nutr, 1997. **77**(4): p. 605-20.

89. Association, A.M., *American Medical Association Essential Guide to Menopause.* 1 ed. 1998, New York: Pocket Books. 253.

90. Jeppesen, J., *et al.*, *Effects of low-fat, high-carbohydrate diets on risk factors for ischemic heart disease in post-menopausal women [published erratum appears in Am J Clin Nutr 1997 Aug;66(2):437].* Am J Clin Nutr, 1997. **65**(4): p. 1027-33.

91. Grundy, S., *Comparison of monounsaturated fatty acids and carbohydrates for lowering plasma cholesterol.* N Eng J Med, 1986. **314**: p. 745-748.

92. Garg, A., *et al.*, *Comparison of a high-carbohydrate diet with a high-monounsaturated-fat diet in patients with non-insulin-dependent diabetes mellitus.* N Engl J Med, 1988. **319**(13): p. 829-34.

93. Bush, T., E. Barrett-Connor, and L. Cowan, *et al.*, *Cardiovascular mortality and noncontraceptive use of estogen in women: results from the Lipid Research Clinics Program Follow-up Study.* Circulation, 1987. **75**: p. 1102-9.

94. Brunner, D., J. Weisbort, and N. Meshulam, *et al.*, *Relation of serum total cholesterol an dhigh-density lipoprotein cholesterol percentage to the incidence of definite coronary events:twenty-year follow-up of the Donolo-Tel Aviv prospective coronary artery disease study.* Am J Cardiol, 1987. **59**: p. 1271-6.

95. Bass, K *et al.*, *Plasma lipoprotein levels as predictors of cardiovascular death in women.* Arch Intern Med, 1993. **153**: p. 2209-16.

96. Stensvold, I., *et al.*, *Non-fasting serum triglyceride concentration and mortality from coronary heart disease and any cause in middle-aged Norwegian women*. Br J Med, 1993. **307**: p. 1318-22.

97. Sugano, M., *Characteristics of fats in Japanese diets and current recommendations*. Lipids, 1996. **31** Suppl: p.S283-6.

98. Weisburger, J.H., *Dietary fat and risk of chronic disease: mechanistic insights from experimental studies*. J Am Diet Assoc, 1997. **97**(7 Suppl): p. S16-23.

99. Masai, M., H. Ito, and T. Kotake, *Effect of dietary intake on urinary oxalate excretion in calcium renal stone formers*. Br J Urol, 1995. **76**(6): p. 692-6.

100. Schwille, P., E. Hanisch, and D. Scholz, *Postprandial hyperoxaluria and intestinal oxalate absorption in idiopathic renal stone disease*. J Urol, 1984. **132**: p. 650-5.

101. Trinchierti, A., *et al.*, *The influence of diet on urinary risk factors for stones in healthy subjects and idiopathic reanl calcium stone formers*. Br J Urol, 1991. **67**: p. 230-6.

102. Curhan, G.C., *et al.*, *Comparison of dietary calcium with supplemental calcium and other nutrients as factors affecting the risk for kidney stones in women [see comments]*. Ann Intern Med, 1997. **126**(7): p. 497-504.

103. Curhan, G.C., *et al.*, *Beverage use and risk for kidney stones in women*. Ann Intern Med, 1998. **128**(7): p. 534-40.

104. Schubert, W., *et al.*, *Inhibition of 17 beta-estradiol metabolism by grapefruit juice in ovariectomized women*. Maturitas, 1994. **20**(2-3): p. 155-63.

105. Lustig, R., R. Hershcopf, and H. Bradlow, *The*

effects of body weight and diet on estrogen metabolism and estrogen-dependent disease, in Adipose Tissue and Reproduction, R. Frisch, Editor. 1990, **Karger**: Basel. p. 107-124.

106. Fishman, J., J. Schneider, and R. Hershcopf, *et al., Increased estrogen 16alpha-hydroxylase activity in women with breast and endometrial cancer.* J Steroid Biochem, 1984. **20**: p. 1077-1081.

107. Bradlow, H., R. Hershcopf, and J. Fishman, *Oestradiol 16 alpha-hydroxylase: a risk marker for breast cancer.* Cancer surv, 1986. **5**: p. 573-583.

108. Munger, R.G., J.R. Cerhan, and B.C. Chiu, *Prospective study of dietary protein intake and risk of hip fracture in postmenopausal women.* Am J Clin Nutr, 1999. **69**(1): p. 147-52.

109. Knight, D.C. and J.A. Eden, *A review of the clinical effects of phytoestrogens.* Obstet Gynecol, 1996. **87**(5 Pt 2): p. 897-904.

110. Arjmandi, B.H., *et al., Role of soy protein with normal or reduced isoflavone content in reversing bone loss induced by ovarian hormone deficiency in rats.* Am J Clin Nutr, 1998. **68**(6 Suppl): p. 1358S-1363S.

111. Challier, B., J.M. Perarnau, and J.F. Viel, *Garlic, onion and cereal fibre as protective factors for breast cancer: a French case-control study.* Eur J Epidemiol, 1998. **14**(8): p. 737-47.

112. Nestel, P.J., *et al., Soy isoflavones improve systemic arterial compliance but not plasma lipids in menopausal and perimenopausal women.* Arterioscler Thromb Vasc Biol, 1997. **17**(12): p. 3392-8.

113. Simon, A.H., *et al., Renal haemodynamic responses to a chicken or beef meal in normal individuals.* Nephrol

Dial Transplant, 1998. **13**(9): p. 2261-4.

114. Anderson, J.W., *et al.*, *Effects of soy protein on renal function and proteinuria in patients with type 2 diabetes.* Am J Clin Nutr, 1998. **68**(6 Suppl): p. 1347S-1353S.

115. Murkies, A., *Phytoestrogens-what is the current knowledge?* Aust. Fam Physician, 1998. **27**(suppl 1): p. 547-551.

116. Ferraroni, M., *et al.*, *Alcohol consumption and risk of breast cancer: a multicentre Italian case-control study [see comments].* Eur J Cancer, 1998. **34**(9): p. 1403-9.

117. Oneta, C., *et al.*, *First pass metabolism of ethanol is strikingly influenced by the speed of gastric emptying.* Gut, 1998. **43**(5): p. 612-9.

118. Ginsburg, E.S., *et al.*, *The effect of acute ethanol ingestion on estrogen levels in postmenopausal women using transdermal estradiol.* J Soc Gynecol Investig, 1995. **2**(1): p. 26-9.

119. Purohit, V., *Moderate alcohol consumption and estrogen levels in postmenopausal women: a review.* Alcohol Clin Exp Res, 1998. **22**(5): p. 994-7.

120. Bradley, K.A., *et al.*, *Medical risks for women who drink alcohol.* J Gen Intern Med, 1998. **13**(9): p. 627-39.

121. Muti, P., *et al.*, *Alcohol consumption and total estradiol in premenopausal women.* Cancer Epidemiol Biomarkers Prev, 1998. **7**(3): p. 189-93.

122. Dallongeville, J., *et al.*, *Influence of alcohol consumption and various beverages on waist girth and waist-to-hip ratio in a sample of French men and women.* Int J Obes Relat Metab Disord, 1998. **22**(12): p. 1178-83.

123. Criqui, M.H., *Do known cardiovascular risk*

factors mediate the effect of alcohol on cardiovascular disease?. Novartis Found Symp, 1998. **216**: p. 159-67.

124. Godfroid, *I.O., Eulogy of wine?.* Presse Med, 1997. **26**(40): p. 1971-4.

125. Lloyd, T., *et al., Dietary caffeine intake and bone status of postmenopausal women.* Am J Clin Nutr, 1997. **65**(6): p. 1826-30.

126. Tavani, A., E. Negri, and C. La Vecchia, *Coffee intake and risk of hip fracture in women in northern Italy.* Prev Med, 1995. **24**(4): p. 396-400.

127. Tavani, A., *et al., Coffee consumption and the risk of breast cancer.* Eur J Cancer Prev, 1998. **7**(1): p. 77-82.

128. Tavani, A., *et al., Coffee and tea intake and risk of cancers of the colon and rectum: a study of 3,530 cases and 7,057 controls.* Int J Cancer, 1997. **73**(2): p. 193-7.

129. Pizziol, A., *et al., Effects of caffeine on glucose tolerance: a placebo-controlled study.* Eur J Clin Nutr, 1998. **52**(11): p. 846-9.

130. Kleiner, S.M., *Water: an essential but overlooked nutrient.* J Am Diet Assoc, 1999. **99**(2): p. 200-6.

131. Svetkey, L.P., *et al., Preliminary evidence of linkage of salt sensitivity in black Americans at the beta 2-adrenergic receptor locus.* Hypertension, 1997. **29**(4): p. 918-22.

132. Chan, T.Y., *et al., Urinary dopamine outputs do not rise in healthy Chinese subjects during gradually increasing oral sodium intake over 8 days.* J Auton Pharmacol, 1996. **16**(3): p. 155-9.

133. Iwaoka, T., *et al., The effect of low and high NaCl diets on oral glucose tolerance.* Klin Wochenschr, 1988. **66**(16): p. 724-8.

134. Gonzalez Vilchez, F., *et al.*, *Cardiac manifestations of primary hypothyroidism. Determinant factors and treatment response.* Rev Esp Cardiol, 1998. **51**(11): p. 893-900.

135. Massoudi, M.S., *et al.*, *Prevalence of thyroid antibodies among healthy middle-aged women. Findings from the thyroid study in healthy women.* Ann Epidemiol, 1995. **5**(3): p. 229-33.

136. Nunez, S. and J. Leclere, *Diagnosis of hypothyroidism in the adult.* Rev Prat, 1998. **48**(18): p. 1993-8.

137. Stockigt, J.R., *Thyroid disease.* Med J Aust, 1993. **158**(11): p. 770-4.

138. Reinhardt, W., *et al.*, *Effect of small doses of iodine on thyroid function in patients with Hashimoto's thyroiditis residing in an area of mild iodine deficiency.* Eur J Endocrinol, 1998. **139**(1): p. 23-8.

139. Konno, N., *et al.*, *Association between dietary iodine intake and prevalence of subclinical hypothyroidism in the coastal regions of Japan.* J Clin Endocrinol Metab, 1994. **78**(2): p. 393-7.

140. Levi, B. and M.J. Werman, *Long-term fructose consumption accelerates glycation and several age- related variables in male rats.* J Nutr, 1998. **128**(9): p. 1442-9.

141. Gannon, M.C., *et al.*, *Stimulation of insulin secretion by fructose ingested with protein in people with untreated type 2 diabetes.* Diabetes Care, 1998. **21**(1): p. 16-22.

142. Okuno, G., *et al.*, *Glucose tolerance, blood lipid, insulin and glucagon concentration after single or continuous administration of aspartame in diabetics.* Diabetes Res Clin Pract, 1986. **2**(1): p. 23-7.

143. Malaisse, W.J., *et al.*, *Effects of artificial sweeteners on*

insulin release and cationic fluxes in rat pancreatic islets. Cell Signal, 1998. **10**(10): p. 727-33.

144. Vezina, W.C., *et al.*, *Similarity in gallstone formation from 900 kcal/day diets containing 16 g vs 30 g of daily fat: evidence that fat restriction is not the main culprit of cholelithiasis during·rapid weight reduction.* Dig Dis Sci, 1998. **43**(3): p. 554-61.

145. Edes, T.E. and J.H. Shah, *Glycemic index and insulin response to a liquid nutritional formula compared with a standard meal.* J Am Coll Nutr, 1998. **17**(1): p. 30-5.

146. Sharma, R.D., T.C. Raghuram, and N.S. Rao, *Effect of fenugreek seeds on blood glucose and serum lipids in type I diabetes.* Eur J Clin Nutr, 1990. **44**(4): p. 301-6.

147. McGinnis, J.M., *The public health burden of a sedentary lifestyle.* Med Sci Sports Exerc, 1992. **24**(6 Suppl): p. S196-200.

148. McTiernan, A., *et al.*, *Prevalence and correlates of recreational physical activity in women aged 50-64 years.* Menopause, 1998. **5**(2): p. 95-101.

149. Visser, M., *et al.*, *Total and sports activity in older men and women: relation with body fat distribution.* Am J Epidemiol, 1997. **145**(8): p. 752-61.

150. Hu, J.F., *et al.*, *Bone density and lifestyle characteristics in premenopausal and postmenopausal Chinese women.* Osteoporos Int, 1994. **4**(6): p. 288-97.

151. Nicklas, B.J., E.M. Rogus, and A.P. Goldberg, *Exercise blunts declines in lipolysis and fat oxidation after dietary-induced weight loss in obese older women.* Am J Physiol, 1997. **273**(1 Pt 1): p. E149-55.

152. Despres, J.P., *et al.*, *Loss of abdominal fat and metabolic response to exercise training in obese women.* Am

J Physiol, 1991. **261**(2 Pt 1): p. E159-67.

153. Buemann, B. and A. Tremblay, *Effects of exercise training on abdominal obesity and related metabolic complications.* Sports Med, 1996. **21**(3): p. 191-212.

154. Lewis, S., *et al., Effects of physical activity on weight reduction in obese middle-aged women.* Am J Clin Nutr, 1976. **29**(2): p. 151-6.

155. Sanborn, C.F. and C.M. Jankowski, *Physiologic considerations for women in sport.* Clin Sports Med, 1994. **13**(2): p. 315-27.

156. Leon, A.S., *et al., Leisure-time physical activity levels and risk of coronary heart disease and death. The Multiple Risk Factor Intervention Trial.* Jama, 1987. **258**(17): p. 2388-95.

157. Ryan, A.S., B.J. Nicklas, and K.E. Dennis, *Aerobic exercise maintains regional bone mineral density during weight loss in postmenopausal women.* J Appl Physiol, 1998. **84**(4): p. 1305-10.

158. Kirk, S., *et al., Effect of long-distance running on bone mass in women.* J Bone Miner Res, 1989. **4**(4): p. 515-22.

159. van Dam, S., *et al., Effect of exercise on glucose metabolism in postmenopausal women.* Am J Obstet Gynecol, 1988. **159**(1): p. 82-6.

160. Baker, C.L., Jr., *Lower extremity problems in female athletes.* J Med Assoc Ga, 1997. **86**(3): p. 193-6.

161. Wojtys, E.M., *et al., Association between the menstrual cycle and anterior cruciate ligament injuries in female athletes.* Am J Sports Med, 1998. **26**(5): p. 614-9.

162. Liu, S.H., *et al., Estrogen affects the cellular metabolism of the anterior cruciate ligament. A potential*

explanation for female athletic injury. Am J Sports Med, 1997. **25**(5): p. 704-9.

163. Ryan, A.S., *et al., Resistive training maintains bone mineral density in postmenopausal women.* Calcif Tissue Int, 1998. **62**(4): p. 295-9.

164. Morganti, C.M., *et al., Strength improvements with 1 yr of progressive resistance training in older women.* Med Sci Sports Exerc, 1995. **27**(6): p. 906-12.

165. Thomas, D.E., J.R. Brotherhood, and J.C. Brand, *Carbohydrate feeding before exercise: effect of glycemic index.* Int J Sports Med, 1991. **12**(2): p. 180-6.

166. Thompson, J.L., *et al., Effects of human growth hormone, insulin-like growth factor I, and diet and exercise on body composition of obese postmenopausal women.* J Clin Endocrinol Metab, 1998. **83**(5): p. 1477-84.

167. Svendsen, O.L., *et al., Effects on muscle of dieting with or without exercise in overweight postmenopausal women.* J Appl Physiol, 1996. **80**(4): p. 1365-70.

168. Wouassi, D., *et al., Metabolic and hormonal responses during repeated bouts of brief and intense exercise: effects of pre-exercise glucose ingestion.* Eur J Appl Physiol, 1997. **76**(3): p. 197-202.

169. Seals, D.R., *et al., Effect of regular aerobic exercise on elevated blood pressure in postmenopausal women.* Am J Cardiol, 1997. **80**(1): p. 49-55.

170. Leitzmann, M.F., *et al., The relation of physical activity to risk for symptomatic gallstone disease in men.* Ann Intern Med, 1998. **128**(6): p. 417-25.

171. Bass, S., *et al., Exercise before puberty may confer residual benefits in bone density in adulthood: studies in active prepubertal and retired female gymnasts.* J Bone

Miner Res, 1998. **13**(3): p. 500-7.

172. Kohrt, W.M., A.A. Ehsani, and S.J. Birge, Jr., *HRT preserves increases in bone mineral density and reductions in body fat after a supervised exercise program.* J Appl Physiol, 1998. **84**(5): p. 1506-12.

173. Kraemer, R.R., *et al.*, *Effects of hormone replacement on growth hormone and prolactin exercise responses in postmenopausal women.* J Appl Physiol, 1998. **84**(2): p. 703-8.

174. Notelovitz, M., *et al.*, *Estrogen therapy and variable-resistance weight training increase bone mineral in surgically menopausal women.* J Bone Miner Res, 1991. **6**(6): p. 583-90.

175. Kritz-Silverstein, D. and E. Barrett-Connor, *Long-term postmenopausal hormone use, obesity, and fat distribution in older women [see comments].* Jama, 1996. **275**(1): p. 46-9.

176. Luoto, R., S. Mannisto, and E. Vartiainen, *Hormone replacement therapy and body size: how much does lifestyle explain?* Am J Obstet Gynecol, 1998. **178**(1 Pt 1): p. 66-73.

177. De Lorenzo, A., *et al.*, *Body composition and androgen pattern in the early period of postmenopause.* Gynecol Endocrinol, 1998. **12**(3): p. 171-7.

178. Simpson, E., *et al.*, *Regulation of estrogen biosynthesis by human adipose cells.* Endoc Rev, 1989. **10**: p. 136-148.

179. Wild, R.A., *et al.*, *Clinical signs of androgen excess as risk factors for coronary artery disease.* Fertil Steril, 1990. **54**(2): p. 255-9.

180. Schillaci, G., *et al.*, *Early cardiac changes after*

menopause. Hypertension, 1998. **32**(4): p. 764-9.

181. Mercuro, G., *et al., Estradiol-17beta reduces blood pressure and restores the normal amplitude of the circadian blood pressure rhythm in postmenopausal hypertension.* Am J Hypertens, 1998. **11**(8 Pt 1): p. 909-13.

182. Phillips, G.B., T.Y. Jing, and J.H. Laragh, *Serum sex hormone levels in postmenopausal women with hypertension.* J Hum Hypertens, 1997. **11**(8): p. 523-6.

183. Sudhir, K., *et al., Estrogen supplementation decreases norepinephrine-induced vasoconstriction and total body norepinephrine spillover in perimenopausal women.* Hypertension, 1997. **30**(6): p. 1538-43.

184. Kaufert, P., *et al., Women and menopause: beliefs, attitudes, and behaviors. The North American Menopause Society 1997 Menopause Survey.* Menopause, 1998. **5**(4): p. 197-202.

185. Newton, K.M., *et al., Women's beliefs and decisions about hormone replacement therapy.* J Womens Health, 1997. **6**(4): p. 459-65.

186. Lydakis, C., *et al., Women's awareness of, and attitudes towards, hormone replacement therapy: ethnic differences and effects of age and education.* Int J Clin Pract, 1998. **52**(1): p. 7-12.

187. France, K., M.J. Schofield, and C. Lee, *Patterns and correlates of hormone replacement therapy use among middle-aged Australian women.* Womens Health, 1997. **3**(2): p. 121-38.

188. Bastion, L., *et al., Perceptions of menopausal status and patterns of hormone replacement therapy use.* J Womens Health, 1997. **6**(4): p. 467-75.

189. Schneider, H.P., *Cross-national study of women's*

use of hormone replacement therapy (HRT) in Europe. Int J Fertil Womens Med, 1997. **42**(Suppl 2): p. 365-75.

190. Oddens, B.J. and M.J. Boulet, *Hormone replacement therapy among Danish women aged 45-65 years: prevalence, determinants, and compliance.* Obstet Gynecol, 1997. **90**(2): p. 269-77.

191. Haines, C.J., et al., *The perception of the menopause and the climacteric among women in Hong Kong and southern China.* Prev Med, 1995. **24**(3): p. 245-8.

192. McNagny, S.E. and T.A. Jacobson, *Use of post-menopausal hormone replacement therapy by African American women. The importance of physician discussion.* Arch Intern Med, 1997. **157**(12): p. 1337-42.

193. Rosenberg, L., et al., *Correlates of postmenopausal female hormone use among black women in the United States.* Obstet Gynecol, 1998. **91**(3): p.454-8.

194. Feher, M.D. and A.J. Isaacs, *Is hormone replacement therapy prescribed for postmenopausal diabetic women?* Br J Clin Pract, 1996. **50**(8): p. 431-2.

195. Brett, K.M. and J.H. Madans, *Use of postmenopausal hormone replacement therapy: estimates from a nationally representative cohort study.* Am J Epidemiol, 1997. **145**(6): p. 536-45.

196. McNagny, S.E., N.K. Wenger, and E. Frank, *Personal use of postmenopausal hormone replacement therapy by women physicians in the United States.* Ann Intern Med, 1997. **127**(12): p. 1093-6.

197. Isaacs, A.J., A.R. Britton, and K. McPherson, *Why do women doctors in the UK take hormone replacement therapy?* J Epidemiol Community Health, 1997. **51**(4): p. 373-7.

198. Frank, E., *et al., Health-related behaviors of women physicians vs other women in the United States.* Arch Intern Med, 1998. **158**(4): p. 342-8.

199. US Department of Health and Human Services, P.H.S., *Center for Disease Control and Prevention, National Center for Health Statistics, Death and Death rates for the 10 leading causes of death in specified age groups, by race and sex: US 1996.* National Vital Statistics Report, 1998. **47**(9): p. 29, 32, 36, 64-65.

200. Marrugat, J., *et al., Mortality differences between men and women following first myocardial infarction. RESCATE Investigators. Recursos Empleados en el Sindrome Coronario Agudo y Tiempo de Espera.* Jama, 1998. **280**(16): p. 1405-9.

201. Gerhard, G., *Premenopausal black women have more risk factors for coronary heart disease than white women.* Am J Cardiol, 1998. **82**: p. 1040-1045.

202. Bailey, J., *et al., HRT and Cardio-Protection: Unravelling the tangled web.* Eur Menopause J, 1997. **4**(1): p. I-IV.

203. Wingrove, C.S. and J.C. Stevenson, *17 beta-Oestradiol inhibits stimulated endothelin release in human vascular endothelial cells.* Eur J Endocrinol, 1997. **137**(2): p. 205-8.

204. Wingrove, C.S., *et al., 17beta-oestradiol enhances release of matrix metalloproteinase-2 from human vascular smooth muscle cells.* Biochim Biophys Acta, 1998. **1406**(2): p. 169-74.

205. Manson, J.E., *Postmenopausal hormone therapy and atherosclerotic disease.* Am Heart J, 1994. **128**(6 Pt 2): p. 1337-43.

206. Cowan, L.D., *et al., Parity, postmenopausal estro-*

gen use, and cardiovascular disease risk factors in American Indian women: the Strong Heart Study. J Womens Health, 1997. **6**(4): p. 441-9.

207. Williams, S., et al., Effect of minocycline on osteoporosis. Adv Dent Res, 1998. **12**(2): p. 71-5.

208. Felson, D.T. and M.C. Nevitt, The effects of estrogen on osteoarthritis. Curr Opin Rheumatol, 1998. **10**(3): p. 269-72.

209. Reinhardt, R.A., et al., Gingival fluid IL-1 beta and IL-6 levels in menopause. J Clin Periodontol, 1994. **21**(1): p. 22-5.

210. Grodstein, F., G. Colditz, and M. Stampfer, Post-menopausal hormone use and tooth loss: a prospective study. J Am Dent Assoc, 1996. **127**(3): p. 370-7.

211. Renfro, J. and J.B. Brown, Understanding and preventing osteoporosis. Aaohn J, 1998. **46**(4): p. 181-91; quiz 192-3.

212. Boning up on Osteoporosis, 1999, National Osteoporosis Foundation.

213. Bason, W., Osteoporosis among estrogen-deficient women - United States, 1988-1994. JAMA, 1999. **281**(3): p. 224-226.

214. Perry, H.M., 3rd, et al., The effect of aging on bone mineral metabolism and bone mass in Native American women. J Am Geriatr Soc, 1998. **46**(11): p. 1418-22.

215. Tobias, J.H., et al., A comparison of bone mineral density between Caucasian, Asian and Afro-Caribbean women. Clin Sci (Colch), 1994. **87**(5): p. 587-91.

216. Elkind-Hirsch, K., E. Wallace, and B. Stach, Cyclic steroid replacement alters auditory brainstem

responses in young women with premature ovarian failure. Hear Res, 1992. **64**: p. 93-98.

217. Ries, P., *Prevalence and characteristics of persons with hearing trouble: United States 1990-01.* Vital Health Stat, 1994. **10**: p. 188.

218. Gates, G., J. Cobb, and D. A. R, *The relation of hearing in the elderly to the presence of cardiovascular disease and cardiovascular risk factors.* Arch Otolaryngol Head Neck Surg, 1993. **119**: p. 156-161.

219. Rosen, S., P. Olin, and H. Rosen, *Dietary prevention of hearing loss.* Acta Otolaryngol, 1970. **70**: p. 242-247.

220. Sator, M.O., *et al., Reduction of intraocular pressure in a glaucoma patient undergoing hormone replacement therapy.* Maturitas, 1998. **29**(1): p. 93-5.

221. Lippert, T.H., *et al., Serotonin metabolite excretion after postmenopausal estradiol therapy.* Maturitas, 1996. **24**(1-2): p. 37-41.

222. Eriksen, B.C. and S. Hunskar, *Urogenital estrogen deficiency syndrome. Investigation and treatment with special reference to hormone substitution.* Tidsskr Nor Laegeforen, 1991. **111**(24): p. 2949-51.

223. Sherwin, B.B., *Estrogen and cognitive functioning in women.* Proc Soc Exp Biol Med, 1998. **217**(1): p. 17-22.

224. Eden, J.A., *Progestogens: an occasional review.* Asia Oceania J Obstet Gynaecol, 1991. **17**(4): p. 289-95.

225. Bardin, C.W., *et al., Progestins can mimic, inhibit and potentiate the actions of androgens.* Pharmacol Ther, 1983. **23**(3): p. 443-59.

226. Kontula, K., *et al., Binding of progestins to the*

glucocorticoid receptor. Correlation to their glucocorticoid-like effects on in vitro functions of human mononuclear leukocytes. Biochem Pharmacol, 1983. **32**(9): p. 1511-8.

227. Ashby, J.P., D. Shirling, and J.D. Baird, *Effect of progesterone on the secretion and peripheral action of insulin and glucagon in the intact rat.* J Endocrinol, 1981. **88**(1): p. 49-55.

228. Hargrove, J., *et al.*, *Menopausal hormone replacement therapy with continuous daily oral micronized estradiol and progesterone.* Obstet Gynecol, 1989. **73**(4): p. 606-12.

229. Ettinger, B., *et al.*, *Low-dosage micronized 17b-estradiol prevents bone loss in postmenopausal women.* Am J Obstet Gynecol, 1992. **166**: p. 479-88.

230. DeLignieres, B., *Hormone replacement therapy compliance and individually adapted doses.* 7th International Congress on Menopause, ed. B. Von Schoultz and C. Christiansen. 1993, Stockholm: Casterton, Parthenon Publishing Group. 59-67.

231. Frishman, G.N., *The hot flash: pathophysiology and treatment.* R I Med, 1995. **78**(5): p. 132-4.

232. Freedman, R.R., *Biochemical, metabolic, and vascular mechanisms in menopausal hot flashes.* Fertil Steril, 1998. **70**(2): p. 332-7.

233. Cignarelli, M., *et al.*, *Biophysical and endocrine-metabolic changes during menopausal hot flashes: increase in plasma free fatty acid and norepinephrine levels.* Gynecol Obstet Invest, 1989. **27**(1): p. 34-7.

234. Meldrum, D.R., *et al.*, *Pituitary hormones during the menopausal hot flash.* Obstet Gynecol, 1984. **64**(6): p.752-6.

235. Guetta, V., *et al.*, *The role of nitric oxide in coronary vascular effects of estrogen in postmenopausal women.* Circulation, 1997. **96**(9): p. 2795-801.

236. Fields, C.E. and R.G. Makhoul, *Vasomotor tone and the role of nitric oxide.* Semin Vasc Surg, 1998. **11**(3): p. 181-92.

237. American Heart Association, *Take charge. A woman's guide to fighting heart disease,* 1997, American Heart Association: Dallas, TX.

238. Castelo-Branco, C., *et al.*, *Facial wrinkling in post-menopausal women. Effects of smoking status and hormone replacement therapy.* Maturitas, 1998. **29**(1):p.75-86.

239. Uhler, M.L., *et al.*, *Comparison of the impact of transdermal versus oral estrogens on biliary markers of gallstone formation in postmenopausal women.* J Clin Endocrinol Metab, 1998. **83**(2): p. 410-4.

240. Xue, H.Z., *Experimental study on the relation of estrogens to gallstone formation.* Chung Hua Wai Ko Tsa Chih, 1989. **27**(11): p. 686-8, 702-3.

241. Kakar, F., N.S. Weiss, and S.A. Strite, *Non-contraceptive estrogen use and the risk of gallstone disease in women.* Am J Public Health, 1988. **78**(5): p. 564-6.

242. Dourakis, S.P. and G. Tolis, *Sex hormonal preparations and the liver.* Eur J Contracept Reprod Health Care, 1998. **3**(1): p. 7-16.

243. Everson, R.B., D.P. Byar, and A.J. Bischoff, *Estrogen predisposes to cholecystectomy but not to stones.* Gastroenterology, 1982. **82**(1): p. 4-8.

244. Petitti, D.B., S. Sidney, and J.A. Perlman, *Increased risk of cholecystectomy in users of supplemental estrogen.* Gastroenterology, 1988. **94**(1): p. 91-5.

245. Ziel, H.K. and W.D. Finkle, *Increased risk of endometrial carcinoma among users of conjugated estrogens.* N Engl J Med, 1975. **293**(23): p. 1167-70.

246. Smith, D.C., *et al., Association of exogenous estrogen and endometrial carcinoma.* N Engl J Med, 1975. **293**(23): p. 1164-7.

247. Collins, J., *et al., Oestrogen use and survival in endometrial cancer.* Lancet, 1980. **2**(8201): p. 961-4.

248. Hulka, B.S., *et al., Predominance of early endometrial cancers after long-term estrogen use.* JAMA, 1980. **244**(21): p. 2419-22.

249. Persson, I., *Cancer risk in women receiving estrogen-progestin replacement therapy.* Maturitas, 1996. **23** Suppl: p. S37-45.

250. Madigan, M.P., *et al., Serum hormone levels in relation to reproductive and lifestyle factors in postmenopausal women (United States).* Cancer Causes Control, 1998. **9**(2): p. 199-207.

251. Persson, I., *et al., Cancer incidence and mortality in women receiving estrogen and estrogen-progestin replacement therapy—long-term follow-up of a Swedish cohort.* Int J Cancer, 1996. **67**(3): p. 327-32.

252. Holli, K., J. Isola, and J. Cuzick, *Low biologic aggressiveness in breast cancer in women using hormone replacement therapy.* J Clin Oncol, 1998. **16**(9): p. 3115-20.

253. Pritchard, K.I., *Estrogen/hormone replacement therapy and the etiology of breast cancer [In Process Citation].* Recent Results Cancer Res, 1998. **152**: p. 22-31.

254. Sellers, T., *et al., The role of hormone replacement therapy in the risk for breast cancer and total mortality in*

women with a family history of breast cancer. Ann Intern med, 1997. **127**(11): p. 973-80.

255. DiSaia, P.J., *Hormone replacement therapy for breast cancer survivors: facts versus fears.* Clin Oncol, 1995. **7**(4): p. 241-5.

256. Foth, D. and J.M. Cline, *Effects of mammalian and plant estrogens on mammary glands and uteri of macaques.* Am J Clin Nutr, 1998. **68**(6 Suppl): p. 1413S-1417S.

257. Ivarsson, T., A.C. Spetz, and M. Hammar, *Physical exercise and vasomotor symptoms in post-menopausal women.* Maturitas, 1998. **29**(2): p. 139-46.

258. Hirata, J.D., *et al.*, *Does dong quai have estrogenic effects in postmenopausal women? A double-blind, placebo-controlled trial.* Fertil Steril, 1997. **68**(6): p. 981-6.

259. Barton, D.L., *et al.*, *Prospective evaluation of vitamin E for hot flashes in breast cancer survivors.* J Clin Oncol, 1998. **16**(2): p. 495-500.

260. Bairey Merz, C.N., *et al.*, *Cardiovascular stress response and coronary artery disease: evidence of an adverse postmenopausal effect in women.* Am Heart J, 1998. **135**(5 Pt 1): p. 881-7.

261. Jiang, W., *et al.*, *Mental stress—induced myocardial ischemia and cardiac events.* Jama, 1996. **275**(21): p. 1651-6.

262. Gullette, E.C., *et al.*, *Effects of mental stress on myocardial ischemia during daily life.* Jama, 1997. **277**(19): p. 1521-6.

263. Matthews, K.A., *et al.*, *Are hostility and anxiety associated with carotid atherosclerosis in healthy postmenopausal women?* Psychosom Med, 1998. **60**(5): p. 633-8.

264. Haan, C.K., *What Can Be Done to Prevent Coronary Heart Disease in Women?* Medscape Womens Health, 1996. **1**(12): p. 5.

265. Paredes, A., et al., *Stress promotes development of ovarian cysts in rats: the possible role of sympathetic nerve activation.* Endocrine, 1998. **8**(3): p. 309-15.

266. Komesaroff, P.A., et al., *Effects of estrogen and estrous cycle on glucocorticoid and catecholamine responses to stress in sheep.* Am J Physiol, 1998. **275**(4 Pt 1): p. E671-8.

267. Marucha, P.T., J.K. Kiecolt-Glaser, and M. Favagehi, *Mucosal wound healing is impaired by examination stress.* Psychosom Med, 1998. **60**(3): p. 362-5.

268. Kiecolt-Glaser, J.K., et al., *Slowing of wound healing by psychological stress.* Lancet, 1995. **346**(8984): p. 1194-6.

269. Virgin, C.E., Jr., et al., *Glucocorticoids inhibit glucose transport and glutamate uptake in hippocampal astrocytes: implications for glucocorticoid neurotoxicity.* J Neurochem, 1991. **57**(4): p. 1422-8.

270. Kim, J.J. and K.S. Yoon, *Stress: metaplastic effects in the hippocampus.* Trends Neurosci, 1998. **21**(12): p. 505-9.

271. Magarinos, A.M., J.M. Verdugo, and B.S. McEwen, *Chronic stress alters synaptic terminal structure in hippocampus.* Proc Natl Acad Sci U S A, 1997. **94**(25): p. 14002-8.

272. Goodman, Y., et al., *Estrogens attenuate and corticosterone exacerbates excitotoxicity, oxidative injury, and amyloid beta-peptide toxicity in hippocampal neurons.* J Neurochem, 1996. **66**(5): p. 1836-44

273. Reiter, R.J., *Melatonin and human reproduction.* Ann Med, 1998. **30**(1): p. 103-8.

274. Van Cauter, E., *Putative roles of melatonin in glucose regulation.* Therapie, 1998. **53**(5): p. 467-72.

275. Scheen, A.J. and E. Van Cauter, *The roles of time of day and sleep quality in modulating glucose regulation: clinical implications.* Horm Res, 1998. **49**(3-4): p. 191-201.

276. Huerta, R., et al., *Symptoms at the menopausal and premenopausal years: their relationship with insulin, glucose, cortisol, FSH, prolactin, obesity and attitudes towards sexuality.* Psychoneuroendocrinology, 1995. **20**(8): p. 851-64.

277. Smith, J.A., *et al., Human nocturnal blood melatonin and liver acetylation status.* J Pineal Res, 1991. **10**(1):p. 14-7.

278. Frank, S.A., *et al., Effects of aging on glucose regulation during wakefulness and sleep.* Am J Physiol, 1995. **269**(6 Pt 1): p. E1006-16.

279. Rosmond, R., *et al., Mental distress, obesity and body fat distribution in middle-aged men.* Obes Res, 1996. **4**(3): p. 245-52.

280. Van Cauter, E., *et al., Sleep, awakenings, and insulin-like growth factor-I modulate the growth hormone (GH) secretory response to GH-releasing hormone.* J Clin Endocrinol Metab, 1992. **74**(6): p. 1451-9.

281. Grunstein, R.R., *et al., Impact of obstructive sleep apnea and sleepiness on metabolic and cardiovascular risk factors in the Swedish Obese Subjects (SOS) Study.* Int J Obes Relat Metab Disord, 1995. **19**(6): p. 410-8.

282. Rosmond, R. and P. Bjorntorp, *Psychiatric ill-health of women and its relationship to obesity and body fat distribution.* Obes Res, 1998. **6**(5): p. 338-45.

283. Bray, G.A. and D.A. York, *The MONA LISA*

hypothesis in the time of leptin. Recent Prog Horm Res, 1998. **53**: p. 95-117.

284. Bylesjo, E.I., K. Boman, and L. Wetterberg, *Obesity treated with phototherapy: four case studies.* Int J Eat Disord, 1996. **20**(4): p. 443-46.

285. Borody, W.L., T.E. Brown, and R.S. Boroditsky, *Dietary fat and calcium intakes of menopausal women.* Menopause, 1998. **5**(4): p. 230-5.

286. Haines, C.J., *et al., Dietary calcium intake in postmenopausal Chinese women.* Eur J Clin Nutr, 1994. **48**(8): p. 591-4.

287. Lau, E.M. and J. Woo, *Nutrition and osteoporosis.* Curr Opin Rheumatol, 1998. **10**(4): p. 368-72.

288. Verhoef, P., *et al., Arteriosclerosis, Thrombosis and Vascular Biology.* 17, 1997. **5**(989-95).

289. Jacob, R.A., *et al., Moderate folate depletion increases plasma homocysteine and decreases lymphocyte DNA methylation in postmenopausal women.* J Nutr, 1998. **128**(7): p. 1204-12.

290. Devine, A., *et al., Effects of zinc and other nutritional factors on insulin-like growth factor I and insulin-like growth factor binding proteins in postmenopausal women.* Am J Clin Nutr, 1998. **68**(1): p. 200-6.

291. Kennedy, K.J., T.M. Rains, and N.F. Shay, *Zinc deficiency changes preferred macronutrient intake in subpopulations of Sprague-Dawley outbred rats and reduces hepatic pyruvate kinase gene expression.* J Nutr, 1998. **128**(1): p. 43-9.

292. Wood, R.J. and J.J. Zheng, *High dietary calcium intakes reduce zinc absorption and balance in humans.* Am J Clin Nutr, 1997. **65**(6): p. 1803-9.

293. Marks, J.W., *et al.*, *Nucleation of biliary cholesterol, arachidonate, prostaglandin E2, and glycoproteins in postmenopausal women.* Gastroenterology, 1997. **112**(4): p. 1271-6.

294. Simon, J.A., *et al.*, *Ascorbic acid supplement use and the prevalence of gallbladder disease. Heart & Estrogen-Progestin Replacement Study (HERS) Research Group.* J Clin Epidemiol, 1998. **51**(3): p. 257-65.

295. Simon, J.A. and E.S. Hudes, *Serum ascorbic acid and other correlates of gallbladder disease among US adults.* Am J Public Health, 1998. **88**(8): p. 1208-12.

296. Simon, J.A., E.S. Hudes, and W.S. Browner, *Serum ascorbic acid and cardiovascular disease prevalence in U.S. adults.* Epidemiology, 1998. **9**(3): p. 316-21.

297. Hall, S.L. and G.A. Greendale, *The relation of dietary vitamin C intake to bone mineral density: results from the PEPI study.* Calcif Tissue Int, 1998. **63**(3): p. 183-9.

298. Schoenen, J., J. Jacquy, and M. Lenaerts, *Effectiveness of high-dose riboflavin in migraine prophylaxis. A randomized controlled trial.* Neurology, 1998. **50**(2): p. 466-70.

299. Kaul, P., *et al.*, *Calculogenic potential of galactose and fructose in relation to urinary excretion of lithogenic substances in vitamin B6 deficient and control rats.* J Am Coll Nutr, 1996. **15**(3): p. 295-302.

300. Bermond, P., *Therapy of side effects of oral contraceptive agents with vitamin B6.* Acta Vitaminol Enzymol, 1982. **4**(1-2): p. 45-54.

301. Graham, I.M., *et al.*, *Plasma homocysteine as a risk factor for vascular disease. The European Concerted Action Project [see comments].* Jama, 1997. **277**(22): p. 1775-81.

302. Johnston, S.M., *et al.*, *Iron deficiency enhances cholesterol gallstone formation.* Surgery, 1997. **122**(2): p. 354-61; discussion 361-2.

303. Steinberg, D., *et al.*, *Beyond cholesterol. Modifications of low-density lipoprotein that increase its atherogenicity.* N Engl J Med, 1989. **320**(14): p. 915-24.

304. Boger, R.H., *et al.*, *Dietary L-arginine and alpha-tocopherol reduce vascular oxidative stress and preserve endothelial function in hypercholesterolemic rabbits via different mechanisms.* Atherosclerosis, 1998. **141**(1): p. 31-43.

305. Brzozowski, T., *et al.*, *Involvement of endogenous cholecystokinin and somatostatin in gastroprotection induced by intraduodenal fat.* J Clin Gastroenterol, 1998. **27**(Suppl 1): p. S125-37.

306. Reckelhoff, J.F., *et al.*, *Long-term dietary supplementation with L-arginine prevents age-related reduction in renal function.* Am J Physiol, 1997. **272**(6 Pt 2): p. R1768-74.

307. Daly, J.M., *et al.*, *Immune and metabolic effects of arginine in the surgical patient.* Ann Surg, 1988. **208**(4): p. 512-23.

308. Giustina, A., *et al.*, *Arginine blocks the inhibitory effect of hydrocortisone on circulating growth hormone levels in patients with acromegaly.* Metabolism, 1993. **42**(5): p. 664-8.

309. Pomerleau, J., *et al.*, *Effect of protein intake on glycaemic control and renal function in type 2 (non-insulin-dependent) diabetes mellitus.* Diabetologia, 1993. **36**(9): p. 829-34.

310. Preuss, H.G., *et al.*, *Effects of diets high in refined carbohydrates on renal ammonium excretion in rats.* Am J Physiol, 1986. **250**(2 Pt 1): p. E156-63

311. Reyes, A.A. and S. Klahr, *Dietary supplementation of L-arginine ameliorates renal hypertrophy in rats fed a high-protein diet.* Proc Soc Exp Biol Med, 1994. **206**(2): p.157-61.

312. Barzel, U.S. and L.K. Massey, *Excess dietary protein can adversely affect bone.* J Nutr, 1998. **128**(6): p. 1051-3.

313. Hansen, C.M., J.E. Leklem, and L.T. Miller, *Vitamin B-6 status indicators decrease in women consuming a diet high in pyridoxine glucoside.* J Nutr, 1996. **126**(10): p. 2512-8.

314. Shaywitz, S., et al., *Effect of estrogen on brain activation patterns in postmenopausal women during working memory tasks.* JAMA, 1999. **281**: p. 1197-1202.

315. Remer, T. and F. Manz, *Potential renal acid load of foods and its influence on urine pH.* J Am Diet Assoc, 1995. **95**(7): p: 791-7.

316. Schairer, C., Lubin, J., Troisi, R. *et al., Menopausal estrogen and estrogen-progestin replacement therapy and breast cancer risk.* JAMA, 2000. **283** (4): 485-491

317. Persson, I., Weiderpass, E., Bergstrom, R. *et al., Risks of breast and endometrial cancer after estrogen and estrogen-progestin replacement therapy.* Cancer Causes Control, 1999. **10**:253-260.

318. Colditz, G., Hankinson, S., Hunter, D. *et al., The use of estrogens and progestins and the risk of breast cancer in postmenopausal women.* NEJM, 1995. **332**: 1589-1593.

index

order form

Give the gift of great health to your loved ones, friends and colleagues
Check your leading bookstore or order here

fax orders:	**telephone orders:**	**e-mail orders:**	**postal orders:**
(310) 471-9041.	Call	orders@	Healthy Life
(please send a	1-(800) 554-3335	menopausediet.	Publications,
copy of this form)	toll free or	com	264 South
	(310) 471-2375 if outside		La Cienega Blvd.,
	the United States and		PMB #1233,
	Canada. *Have your credit*		Beverly Hills,
	card ready.		California 90211
			USA

Please send _____ copies of *The Menopause Diet* at $17.95 plus $4 shipping per book in the United States (California residents please add $1.48 sales tax per book). Canadian orders must be accompanied by a postal order in U.S. funds. International orders add $9 for shipping.

Please send me information on your other products _____

If you would like to order Female Formula Stress Tabs, Pyridoxal-5-Phosphate or the *Menopause Diet Mini Meal Cookbook,* call 1-800-554-3335 24 hours a day. Operators are waiting for your call.

My check or money order for $_____ is enclosed.
United States $21.95 (outside of California)
                      $23.43 (within California)
Canada $25.00 (US funds)
International $27.00 (US funds)

Please charge my   VISA   MC

Name: _____

Address: _____

City: _____ State: _____ Zip: _____

Phone: _____ E-mail: _____

Card #: _____ Exp date: _____

Signature: _____

Please make your check payable and return to:
Healthy Life Publications
264 S. La Cienega Blvd., PMB #1233, Beverly Hills, California 90211
CALL YOUR CREDIT CARD ORDER TO: 800-554-3335
Fax: 310-471-9041 e-mail: orders@menopausediet.com

order form

Give the gift of great health to your loved ones, friends and colleagues
Check your leading bookstore or order here

fax orders:	**telephone orders:**	**e-mail orders:**	**postal orders:**
(310) 471-9041.	Call	orders@	Healthy Life
(please send a	1-(800) 554-3335	menopausediet.	Publications,
copy of this form)	toll free or	com	264 South
	(310) 471-2375 if outside		La Cienega Blvd.,
	the United States and		PMB #1233,
	Canada. *Have your credit*		Beverly Hills,
	card ready.		California 90211
			USA

Please send _____ copies of *The Menopause Diet* at $17.95 plus $4 shipping per book in the United States (California residents please add $1.48 sales tax per book). Canadian orders must be accompanied by a postal order in U.S. funds. International orders add $9 for shipping.

Please send me information on your other products _____

If you would like to order Female Formula Stress Tabs, Pyridoxal-5-Phosphate or the *Menopause Diet Mini Meal Cookbook*, call 1-800-554-3335 24 hours a day. Operators are waiting for your call.

My check or money order for $_____ is enclosed.
United States $21.95 (outside of California)
                     $23.43 (within California)
Canada $25.00 (US funds)
International $27.00 (US funds)

Please charge my   VISA   MC

Name: _____

Address: _____

City: _____ State: _____ Zip: _____

Phone: _____ E-mail: _____

Card #: _____ Exp date: _____

Signature: _____

Please make your check payable and return to:
Healthy Life Publications
264 S. La Cienega Blvd., PMB #1233, Beverly Hills, California 90211
CALL YOUR CREDIT CARD ORDER TO: 800-554-3335
Fax: 310-471-9041   e-mail: orders@menopausediet.com

Give the gift of great health to your loved ones, friends and colleagues
Check your leading bookstore or order here

fax orders:
(310) 471-9041.
(please send a
copy of this form)

telephone orders:
Call
1-(800) 554-3335
toll free or
(310) 471-2375 if outside
the United States and
Canada. *Have your credit*
card ready.

e-mail orders:
orders@
menopausediet.
com

postal orders:
Healthy Life
Publications,
264 South
La Cienega Blvd.,
PMB #1233,
Beverly Hills,
California 90211
USA

Please send _____ copies of *The Menopause Diet* at $17.95 plus $4 shipping per book in the United States (California residents please add $1.48 sales tax per book). Canadian orders must be accompanied by a postal order in U.S. funds. International orders add $9 for shipping.

Please send me information on your other products _____

If you would like to order Female Formula Stress Tabs, Pyridoxal-5-Phosphate or the *Menopause Diet Mini Meal Cookbook*, call 1-800-554-3335 24 hours a day. Operators are waiting for your call.

My check or money order for $_____ is enclosed.
United States $21.95 (outside of California)
                 $23.43 (within California)
Canada $25.00 (US funds)
International $27.00 (US funds)

Please charge my   VISA   MC

Name: _____

Address: _____

City: _____ State: _____ Zip: _____

Phone: _____ E-mail: _____

Card #: _____ Exp date: _____

Signature: _____

Please make your check payable and return to:
Healthy Life Publications
264 S. La Cienega Blvd., PMB #1233, Beverly Hills, California 90211
CALL YOUR CREDIT CARD ORDER TO: 800-554-3335
Fax: 310-471-9041 e-mail: order@menopausediet.com